I0786539

If you think you've read these blogs before, you're right. As I learned about writing and formatting my books of blogs, I realized *The Book of Blogs: Moderate Stage Chronic Kidney Disease, Parts 1 and 2* were unwieldy to hold and the type was too small. I vowed to correct that. *Part 1* has already been separated into two books: *SlowItDownCKD 2011* and *SlowItDownCKD 2012*.

It seemed to take me forever to get to *Part 2* with life constantly getting in the way. Sure, a lot of that delay was for unwanted reasons like the medical conditions that were uncovered in my family and the deaths, but so much of it was good like the birth of my grandson, our travels, and the marriages of two of our daughters. Life is wonderfully complex that way.

The book series was begun after my family doctor told me I probably had a problem and it had to do with my kidneys, maybe Chronic Kidney Disease. My first reaction was to demand in no uncertain terms, "What is it and how did I get it?" Hence, my first book.

There are many, many of us out there. By us, I mean those who have Chronic Kidney Disease. Friends, partners, family of CKD patients can all gain insight into the daily travails of living with the disease via the blog (SlowItDownCKD) and the books of the same name based on it. I am no expert, but I have tried to read every book I could lay my hands on concerning this disease. Of course, most medical texts are not included because I couldn't understand them. Most of the kidney disease cookbooks aren't included because I can understand a heavy duty medical text better than I can a cookbook. I even read memoirs and biographies to glean what information I could.

Surprisingly, very few of these books dealt with the early or moderate stages of the disease. These are the stages when we, as patients, are most shocked, confused, depressed and at sea. I didn't want to read about transplants or kidney failure. They scared me and I just wasn't ready to learn about them. But I did want to know what was happening to me on a daily basis, what the medications that were ordered for me were supposed to do, and what new discoveries there were that might help slow down this deterioration of my kidneys. That's what the blog and the books are about.

The more you know about Chronic Kidney Disease and the more you read about other people's relationship with it, the more comfortable you'll feel in the early or moderate stages of having the disease yourself. I wish someone had blogged about it when it was new to me. As emails came in asking for print copies of the blogs for those who are not computer savvy or unable to gain access to a computer, I responded by publishing these books of blogs.

I've discovered I have something like 17,000 readers in 109 countries and they're not afraid to tell me what they need to know. I research for them and respond with a blog post, but remind them they need to speak with their nephrologist and/or renal nutritionist before taking any action since I am not a doctor.

I did write several previous books about Chronic Kidney Disease that you'll find referenced many times in the blogs. Those books are **What Is It and How Did I Get It? Early Stage Chronic Kidney Disease** and the other books in the **SlowItDownCKD** series. Each book is the series consists of the blogs for one year. You can find them in print and digital on both Amazon.com and B&N.com. or you can walk into a Barnes and Noble and order them.

I began writing the blog after a doctor in India contacted me telling me he wanted his patients to have the first book, but sometimes they couldn't even afford the bus fare to the clinic. I suggested I start the blog - not having a clue how to do that - he translate it, then print it and give it to patients. The idea was that those who could make it to the clinic would bring the printed copies of the blog back to their villages.

In the interest of keeping the book from becoming mammoth (again), I have omitted the blogs about websites, services, or products that are no longer available. Also omitted were sites that require membership and pay-for-use sites.

I've removed the pictures and a great many references to what was happening at that time in my personal life. I also removed my signature line: "Until next week, keep living your life!" After all, how many times can you read the same sentence in a single book?

When that still didn't shorten the books enough, I removed all notices of past book signings, book talks, Twitter chats, interviews, radio shows, and articles that I'd been involved with. You can't very well go back to the past, so why include them I reasoned.

When you see a set of braces rather than quotation marks, it's me inserting my thoughts into an article.

Welcome to *SlowItDownCKD 2013.*

Keep living your life,
Gail

p.s. As always, I want Bear to know how much I appreciate his respecting Monday as blog day, and when I'm writing a book, Monday, Tuesday, Wednesday, Thursday, Friday, Saturday, and Sunday as writing days. You're one of a kind, honey.

Let The Sun Shine…

1/7/13 Here we are in lovely, warm, sunny Florida. But you just left lovely, warm, sunny Arizona, you may say and you'd be right. Oh, right, hot weather and CKD. The rules for CKD patients in potentially hot weather are the same anywhere in the world.

According to National Kidney Foundation spokesperson,

"Heat illness occurs when body temperature exceeds a person's ability to dissipate that heat and is commonly diagnosed when the body temperature approaches 104 degrees Fahrenheit and when humidity is greater than 70 percent. Once the humidity is that high, sweating becomes less effective at dispersing body heat, and the core body temperature begins to rise."

Now's the time to wear the hat you {meaning I} bought for just that purpose, but forgot was in the trunk of the car. Otherwise, melanoma just might be a possible drawback of a day in the sun.

Melanoma.com tells us:

"Melanoma is the most serious type of skin cancer. It begins in skin cells called melanocytes. Though melanoma is predominantly found on the skin, it can even occur in the eye (uveal melanoma).

Melanocytes are the cells that make melanin, which gives skin its color. Melanin also protects the deeper layers of the skin from the sun's harmful ultraviolet (UV) rays.

When people spend time in the sunlight, the melanocytes make more melanin and cause the skin to tan. This also happens when skin is exposed to other forms of ultraviolet light (such as in a tanning booth). If the skin receives too much ultraviolet light, the melanocytes may begin to grow abnormally and become cancerous."

You are not only heating up your body by being out in hot weather, but exposing yourself to the sun's ultraviolet light. Use that hat to shade some of your body.

DaVita reminds us to use sunscreen with at least 15 SPF. Don't forget if you're swimming – which this aqua-phobe won't be, although I'm looking forward to walking on the beach – you need to slather more on after each dip. You can read more of their hot weather tips, some for dialysis patients, on their website.

You know you need to drink water during hot weather, but is there a difference among waters? Yes, there is. As a CKD patient, your fluid intake is probably restricted {Mine is 64 oz. which includes coffee, tea, juice, ice cream, sherbet, and Jell-O. You get the picture: anything liquid or liquid in a frozen or jelled form.}

Mary Ellen Herndon, a renal nutritionist, warns us

"Many drinks labeled as water are loaded with sugar and empty calories. Even though these drinks have 'water' in their name, drinking them regularly may cause weight gain and may **increase your risk of obesity**."

According to WebMD, we also need to be careful about exercising during the hot weather. I don't mean stop; simply make certain you are not becoming dehydrated. Stay away from energy drinks! As an older adult, I've become aware that I can dehydrate more easily when I exercise – especially since my kidneys are not working at top capacity.

Don't be intimidated by the sun. We can benefit from the sun if we're cautious about it. Fifteen minutes or so a day of sunshine can elevate your vitamin D naturally. Wearing a shirt to cover some of your body can help you protect yourself from the ultraviolet rays while you're indulging in some free vitamin D production.

Be sure to protect your eyes, too.

This is a direct quote from DaVita.

"Sunglasses protect your eyes in the same way that sunscreen protects your skin from harmful sun damage. Your sunglasses should block at least 99% of UVB rays and 50% of UVA rays. Wraparound sunglasses and other styles that completely cover the eyes are best."

By Request, Ladies and Gentlemen: The Flu (Redux)

1/14/13   All around me, I heard coughing, sneezing, throat clearing and sniffling… lots of it. Was this the flu?

That got me to thinking more about the flu just as it was requested that I re-run the flu blogs. Before doing so, I thought I'd find out more about this season's flu. Sure enough, Medpage Today ran just such an article on January 10th of this new year.

"Last week, the CDC reported that 41 states had widespread influenza activity, and 29 states and New York City had high influenza-like illness activity in the week ending Dec. 29. Although not unprecedented, that level of activity is not usually seen until later in the season."

Some of the physicians quoted in the article wondered if it's the reporting of the illness that's improved thereby making the flu appear more widespread than it really is. I don't think I believe that since there seems to be a shortage of both vaccines and drugs to treat this ailment and Boston's mayor has declared a public health emergency due to the 700 cases reported in his city.

According to Healthfinder.gov, you can protect yourself from the flu by doing the following.

"Getting the flu vaccine is the most important step in protecting yourself from the flu. Here are some other things you can do to keep from getting and spreading the flu.

- Stay away from people who are sick.
- If you are sick, stay home for at least 24 hours after your fever is gone.
- Wash your hands often with soap and warm water.
- Try not to touch your nose, mouth, or eyes.
- Cover your mouth and nose with a tissue when you cough or sneeze"

I wondered how to tell the difference between a cold and the flu. Since being diagnosed with CKD, I make it a point to take the flu vaccine annually, yet there have been times when I just didn't feel that well. I found my answer at ABC News.

"With influenza you might also feel very poorly, with aches and pains in your muscles and joints," said Dr. William Schaffner, chair of preventive medicine at Vanderbilt University Medical Center in Nashville, Tenn.

"There's often a cough, too, which is much more prolonged and pronounced. "

I'm including part of an article by The National Kidney Foundation so you can feel confident that your kidneys are being covered here.

"Flu Season and Your Kidneys
By Leslie Spry, MD FACP FASN

As flu season approaches, kidney patients need to know what they can do and what they should avoid if they become ill. The first and most important action to take is to get a flu shot. All patients with Chronic Kidney Disease, including those with a kidney transplant should have a flu shot. Transplant patients may not have the nasal mist flu vaccine known as FluMist®. Transplant patients should have the regular injection for their flu vaccine. If you are a new transplant recipient, within the first 6 months, it is advisable to check with your transplant coordinator to make sure your transplant team allows flu shots in the first 6 months after transplant. ALL other kidney patients should receive a flu vaccination.

If the influenza virus is spreading in your community, there are medications that you can take to protect against influenza if you have not been vaccinated, however the dose of these medications may have to be modified for your level of kidney function. This is also true of antibiotics or any medication that you take for colds, bacterial infections or other viral infections. {I have written about this in both ***What Is It and How Did I Get It? Early Stage Chronic Kidney Disease*** and the blog. You have to tell the prescribing physician about your CKD and/or remind him of it if (s)he already knows each time a prescription is written for you.} The doses of those medications may have to be modified for your level of kidney function. Even if you are vaccinated, it is still possible to get influenza and pneumonia, but the disease is usually much milder.

You should get plenty of rest and avoid other individuals who are ill, in order to limit the spread of the disease. If you are ill, stay home and rest. You should drink plenty of fluids {Remember your limit on fluid intake.} to stay well hydrated. You should eat a balanced diet. If you have gastrointestinal illness including nausea, vomiting or diarrhea, you should contact your physician. Immodium® is generally safe to take to control diarrhea. If you become constipated, medications that contain polyethylene glycol, such as Miralax® and Glycolax® are safe to take. {I've gotten other advice about those brands, so check with your nephrologist before you take anything.} You should avoid laxatives that contain magnesium and phosphates.

Gastrointestinal illness can lead to dehydration or may keep you from taking your proper medication. If you are on a diuretic, it may not be a good idea to keep taking that diuretic if you are unable to keep liquids down or if you are experiencing diarrhea. You should monitor your temperature and blood pressure carefully and report concerns to your physician. Any medication you take should be reported to your physician.

Medications to avoid include all non-steroidal medications including ibuprofen, Motrin®, Advil®, Aleve®, and naproxen. Acetaminophen (Tylenol® and others) and aspirin are generally safe to take with kidney disease. Acetaminophen doses should not exceed 4000 milligrams per day {Nobody ever told me that! Why?} If you take any of the over-the-counter medications, you should always drink plenty of water and stay well hydrated. If you take anti-histamines or decongestants, you should avoid those that contain ephedrine or pseudoephedrine. Over-the-counter cold remedies that are safe to take for patients with high blood pressure are generally designated "HBP". Any over-the-counter medication that you take for a cold or flu should be approved by your doctor."

Again, although this is from a nationally respected doctor, he is not your doctor. Check everything you plan to take with your nephrologist BEFORE you take it. By the way, Medicare covers the cost of the flu shot. Here is some of the information England's Department of Health offered in 2011.

**"Seasonal flu vaccination: Who should have it and why
What harm can seasonal flu do?**

People sometimes think a bad cold is flu, but having flu can be much worse than a cold and you may need to stay in bed for a few days if you have flu. Some people are more susceptible to the effects of seasonal flu. For them it can increase the risk of developing more serious illnesses such as bronchitis and pneumonia, or can make existing conditions worse. In the worst cases, seasonal flu can result in a stay in hospital, or even death.

Am I at greater risk from the effects of seasonal flu?

Even if you feel healthy, you should definitely consider having the free {In England, that is} seasonal flu vaccination if you have:

- a heart problem
- a chest complaint or breathing difficulties, including bronchitis or emphysema
- ***a kidney disease*** {I bolded and italicized this for obvious reasons.}
- lowered immunity due to disease or treatment (such as steroid medication or cancer treatment)
- a liver disease
- had a stroke or a transient ischaemic attack (TIA)
- diabetes
- a neurological condition, for example multiple sclerosis (MS) or cerebral palsy
- a problem with your spleen, for example sickle cell disease, or you have had your spleen removed."

The Flu: Part 3, The Last

1/21/13 Today is such a momentous day. It is not only Martin Luther King, Jr. Day, but the second inauguration of President Obama. As I sit at my computer, I ruminate how far we've come in a relatively short amount of time.

And now I wonder how to slide into a blog about Chronic Kidney Disease. There is no sedge way here. That's all right, though, because we're not exactly dealing with CKD today, but the flu instead. I do promise that this will be the last blog about the flu {this year, that is}. I have just spent four uncomfortable days zapped of energy and not enjoying the movies I watched or books I read while enduring the flu. I was truly surprised at the OTC {Over the counter} medications my nephrologist recommended to me. Tylenol Cold? A steady regime for four days? This for a CKD patient who has taken six Tylenol in the last five years? But that's what the man said.

Dylsem Cough Suppression was another OTC he recommended. Then there was the Benedryl that came with a caution not to take it until I was going to sleep. It would knock me out. Oh, and the Mucinex. The one recommendation I got a kick from was hot tea with lemon and honey laced with whiskey. This for someone who doesn't drink?

Now that I'm feeling better – even if I don't sound better – I'm nervous about all this medication. I carefully read each and every label. Not a single one mentioned anything about possible kidney damage.

I think I've become accustomed to not taking OTC medication and I think that's done me well. As I finished each bottle of medication – especially the Tylenol Cold – I noticed I felt more alert, more aware of my body, and less... less what? Tamped down? Cocooned? I don't know the word, but I certainly feel more here.

Is it that the medications did their job? Probably. Is it that I got more sleep and rest than I have in quite a while? Probably that, too. But maybe, just maybe, my body doesn't like more medications. Sounds a bit hocus-pocus, but this is the same body that has slowly raised its GFR with careful guidance from me.

Would I take the flu shot again even though I got the flu after taking it this season? Absolutely. It was my misfortune to take the immunization for the wrong strain of flu this year. That's never happened before, but then again, there haven't usually been this many different strains of flu before in the same season.

Another reason is that this inoculation against influenza also prevents heart attack and stroke.

"If you're tempted to skip your flu shot, consider this: Getting vaccinated cuts risk for a heart attack or stroke by up to 50 percent, according to two studies presented at the Canadian Cardiovascular Congress."

That was the lead sentence in Lisa Collier Cool's Nov. 26, 2012 Yahoo Health article.

According to a Reuters' Jan. 18, 2013 article, the number of flu cases is beginning to taper off but this has been a difficult year. We already know that. Both Boston and New York State have declared Medical Health Emergencies. Look around you. Are there people missing from your office? Your school? I noticed fewer people in the markets, too. This same article talks about a dearth of Tamiflu. Weren't we told just last week that there was a shortage of the vaccine, too? Do you see where I'm going with this? If you haven't gotten your inoculation, get it. If you have, but can't find Tamiflu {not that everyone is prescribed Tamiflu}, ask your doctor. No reason to panic. Honestly, I sometimes wonder just how objective our news is.

A Medpage Today article offered some startling information on January 19th of this year.

"A resounding 85% of 2,000-plus *Medpage Today* readers voted 'yes' to our survey question asking if media attention promoted a 'pseudo epidemic' as patients mistake cold symptoms for flu."

Did I do that? Did you? As someone who rarely becomes ill for more than a day at a time, did I simply not recognize a bad cold for what it is?

I couldn't secure an appointment with my PCP {primary care physician} until this coming Wednesday – fully a week after I started to feel symptoms. Will it be too late for her to tell the difference?

As I read a New York Times article about the severe flu season from last Saturday, it occurred to me that when the media refers to the elderly, they mean people over 65. That means me! I had not been paying attention to any health warnings for the elderly because they didn't apply to me. Hah! Reality smacks me in the face again.

Back To Basics

1/28/13   I chose communication about CKD as the topic for this week's blog because I have been doing just that… and being startled over and over again at the number of people I've spoken with that know nothing about Chronic Kidney Disease. So, this week, we go back to basics.

Anyone know what the kidneys are and what they do? Will the gentleman with his hand raised in the back of the room answer the question, please? Oh, it's my future son-in-law and he's quoting me! On page 1 of ***What Is It and How Did I Get It? Early Stage Chronic Kidney Disease***, I wrote,

"Later, I learned that the kidneys were two reddish brown organs which lay on the muscles of the back on either side of your spine above hipbone level and below the diaphragm… Some have compared their size to that of a clenched fist or a large computer mouse, and the right one lies lower than the left since the liver is on that side."

Now about their function… Ah, lady on the left side of the room. My dear East Coast buddy, I didn't know you were here.

According to The National Kidney and Urologic Diseases Information Clearinghouse (NKUDIC), A service of **the** National Institute of Diabetes and Digestive and Kidney Diseases (NIDDK)**,**

"Every day, a person's kidneys process about 200 quarts of blood to sift out about 2 quarts of waste products and extra water. The wastes and extra water become urine, which flows to the bladder through tubes called ureters. The bladder stores urine until releasing it through urination."

Nice job! What else do they do? Nima? Yes, you may answer questions even though you're my daughter. Well then.

- Control your body's chemical balance
- Help control your blood pressure
- Help keep your bones healthy
- Help you make red blood cells

You've learned well. What was your source? Glad to hear it was The American Kidney Fund.

That's a good one, as are all the others mentioned here. They each contain far more information than we've included in today's blog and can make you a sort of neophyte kidney expert. Well, maybe someone who knows about his/her early stage Chronic Kidney Disease or that of someone you know and/or love might be a more realistic title.

More? Okay. How many people have Chronic Kidney Disease? Look there. Amy, who is in very good health, is here. Ummm, I did tell you that number a few years ago, but it's changed a bit since then. It's 26 million in the USA alone and rising. Those are the diagnosed people. There are millions of other who have not yet realized they have CKD according to The National Kidney Foundation.

How do you know if you have it? Excellent question. As another healthy person, my daughter Abby has asked an important question. Since there are rarely symptoms, it's all about blood and urine tests. A simply stated eHow article explains without overwhelming. Basically, your doctor is looking for protein in your urine and at the following values in your blood test: GFR {glomerular filtration rate} and bun {blood urea nitrogen}.

I will, Bear, right now. He's asked me to make certain I write about the renal diet. He follows it with me so we don't have to cook two different meals.

The renal diet is only one part of the treatment. There's also exercise, adequate sleep and lack of stress. I thought the diet at Buzzle was a good example until I realized there was no potassium restriction on this diet. I follow that of the Northern Arizona Council of Renal Dietitians. What this tells us is that you need to pay attention to the specific renal diet the nephrologist {kidney and high blood pressure expert} has given you or your loved one, friend, and/or co-worker.

"Basically, sodium, phosphorous, protein, potassium and fluids are restricted. Sometimes, I feel like my fluids are exaggerated rather than restricted – like when I'm writing – and have to remind myself to drink so I can meet my 64 ounces/per day 'limit.'"

My neighbor just asked me to backtrack a bit and discuss the causes of CKD. That would be helpful, wouldn't it?

eMedicine explains this well. Two thirds of CKD is caused by high blood pressure or diabetes, but they neglected to mention that sometimes CKD is simply a result of growing older – as in my case.

Frustrated and Wondering

2/4/13 You've seen it all over the *SlowItDownCKD*'s **Facebook page** and on **Twitter**, yesterday was my birthday, my 66th birthday to be exact. But what does my, uh, advanced age mean to my kidneys?

According to my nephrologist, I would lose 1/2 % of my kidney function each year since I was older. Interesting… and wrong. I've gained between 9 and 21 points on my GFR in the last five years. It does vary depending on numerous factors: diet, sleep, exercise, stress, illness. I had my blood drawn two weeks ago and the results told me that my GFR was 52, down from the 64 it had been only three months before. My primary care doctor told me not to worry about this lower number since I had clearly been incubating the flu at the time of the blood draw.

Here's something you haven't heard from me in a while {She wrote tongue in cheek.} that got me to thinking. What do illness – other than Chronic Kidney Disease – and age have to do with your Glomerular Filtration Rate, a widely accepted indication of just how well your kidneys are functioning?

I found the following chart on The National Kidney Foundation's website.

Average Measured GFR by Age in People Without CKD

AGE (Years)	Average Measured GFR (mL/min/1.73 m2)
20-29	116
30-39	107
40-49	99
50-59	93
60-69	85
70+	75

Notice this is for people without CKD.   Now I'm not a mathematician, as we all know, but if those without our disease lose almost ten points of their GFR each decade they age, why am I not surprised that we who do have Chronic Kidney Disease are expected to be lose the same number of points?

By the way, that does take into account the 1/2% a year I would be losing on my GFR – according to my nephrologist – due to age. But it's just not happening.

I have been researching for hours and the only answers I've found to the question of how the flu affected my GFR were on forums or pay-an-expert-for-a-medical-answer sites.

Sorry, folks, I just don't trust them. I will be seeing my nephrologist this week and will make it a point to ask him.

When I had the flu, my nephrologist told me to go right ahead and take the over the counter medications my primary physician had suggested and in the dosages recommended on the labels. He did caution that I not take anything with the letter 'D' in the name since that might raise my blood pressure.

Here's what DaVita has to say about that.

"When the flu season hits, the use of treatments for cold and flu soars. These medications often include compounds that can intensify hypertension and salt retention. Should you require a product to treat cold and/or flu symptoms, it is strongly recommended that you take them as prescribed by your doctor and carefully read the package instructions."

Notice we still don't know if the flu affects the GFR. Although, logically, if hypertension {high blood pressure} affects your kidneys and these medications may raise your blood pressure... perhaps that means they lower your GFR?

These are the kinds of questions that sent me running to interview different nephrologists, rather than trying to research my answers on the internet, when I was writing ***What Is It and How Did I Get it? Early Stage Chronic Kidney Disease***.

I certainly do not mean to beg the issue, but I'm getting nowhere looking for definitive answers as to how my age and any other illness such as the flu affect CKD.

We can all see how age and illness affect us as far as appearance, physical use of our body, and even shrinkage {Proof: I am ½ inch shorter due to the compression of the discs between my vertebrae.}, as well as the coughing, sneezing, and body aches of the flu.

Apparently, you have to be a doctor, or have the vocabulary of one, to be able to understand the connection of these conditions to your GFR.

Whatever Happened To Integrity?

2/11/13   I have been thinking a lot about integrity – or the lack thereof – in today's society. I run into it constantly.

Since this is a blog about Chronic Kidney Disease, you're probably asking yourself, "Okay, so what does this have to do with me?" You, or someone you know and love, just might be out of integrity with themselves about taking care of their CKD and keeping that GFR on the rise.

For example, both my nephrologist and my primary care doctor have been telling me for months that my A1C is too high. That's the blood test that lets you know how your body is handling glucose over a three month period. I politely nodded and said I'd work on it.

But I didn't. I was out of integrity with myself and, if I didn't get right with myself, I was in for trouble in the form of diabetes. We all know how the combination of CKD and diabetes heightens your chances for some kind of cardiovascular event.

This time, I immediately transformed by ceasing to eat any sweets and cutting down my daily carbohydrate intake to between four and six units a day. Think of a unit as a slice of bread or 1/3 cup of spaghetti.
The transforming part is that I don't crave my husband's sweets, even if he's eating them right in front of me. I don't think I've ever been like this before.

My downfall is usually the carbohydrates. I have not gone over my limit once since I decided to become in integrity with myself. I've thought about it and decided it's just not worth it. By the way, I got a little reward for this transformation: my weight dropped immediately and continues to drop.

Maybe it's exercise for you. Are you telling yourself that you'll exercise tomorrow? Is there some guilt in not doing what you need to for your health? We don't just need exercise because we're human; we especially need exercise because we have Chronic Kidney Disease.

Ah, maybe you're one of those people who tell yourself you'll get a good night's sleep tomorrow night, or after you finish that good book, or another project. Doesn't work that way, folks. You can't make up for sleep you missed and we, as those who have CKD, need that sleep.

Or stress? How about stress? I just gave my notice at a job I took because I loved it. Thank goodness, I didn't need the money, but I wasn't ready to retire from this field yet. The last month or so has been so stressful that even I noticed the black rings under my eyes and my inability to remember things clearly enough.

I had to make this right with myself. Once I ascertained that another person could slip right into my place and made arrangements to give her the material she needed, I resigned. Yes, I loved that job but my health is more important. My supervisor is a person of integrity and completely understood the reasons for my resignation.

I Showed You Mine, Now Show Me Yours

2/18/13 I'm starting to wonder what my Chronic Kidney Disease – newly diagnosed as stage 3A or the beginning part of stage 3 – means to our life together. Bear is already wonderful about sharing meals with me when we go out and being sure to order only what I can eat. He even picks up my exercise habit every so often and accepts that I get tired for no reason {Hah!} sometimes. But I suspect there's more.

According to The *Journal of the American Society of Nephrology {JASN}*, a new study reveals your lifetime risk of developing kidney failure.

"Approximately 1 in 40 men and 1 in 60 women of middle age will develop kidney failure if they live into their 90s. People with reduced kidney function face an even higher risk. Kidney failure is on the rise and currently afflicts 2 million people worldwide."

I'm a person with reduced kidney function. So I face a higher than 1 in 60 women risk for kidney failure. Not on your life!!! Or maybe I should say my life.

I'm perfectly capable of keeping that heightened risk at bay and I intend to. I have so much to look forward to. Obviously, we won't be starting a family, but there are daughters, lots of daughters, and they may choose to have their own children – our grandchildren - someday.

Abby is starting her new job today. I wouldn't have missed that for the world. How many better and better positions is she going to find in her career? One couple will have their own wedding next year and I'll be there. I want to see more of Nima… New York isn't that far away. And Lara, how will she choose to have her life develop?

So, you ask, "How will you do that, Gail?" I'll educate myself about Chronic Kidney Disease even more, that's how.

These are the groups I follow on twitter that have information to help me {and you}:

Am Soc Nephrology@ASNKidney – ASN: Leading the Fight Against Kidney Disease.

American Kidney Fund@KidneyFund – The American Kidney Fund fights kidney disease through direct financial support to patients in need, health education and prevention efforts.

DaVita Kidney Care@DaVita – Giving life to dialysis patients. Creating **#kidneyaware** communities. Cultivating leadership with **#davitau**. Living our core value of fun.

Joel Topf @kidney_boy – Salt whisperer, nephrologist, runner, blogger and editor of **@kidometer**. Interests: teaching, medicine, electrolytes, CKD, and all things Apple **#FOAMed** advocate

Kidney Foundation@ChattanoogaKF – To provide help and information to those affected by kidney disease.

Mostly Medical Links@MostlyMedLinks – Interesting medical news and links via **@JoshuaSchwimmer**, a nephrologist.

NurseGroups@NurseGroups – The social career resource for nurses. Tweeting daily nursing and health news. **#Team Nurses**

NYTimes Health@nytimeshealth – Health news from the Science desk of The New York Times

Renal Info@renalinfo – Baxter is a diversified company that develops & manufactures products that save and sustain the lives of people with kidney disease and other medical conditions

RNCentral.com @RNCentral - Nursing education, news, and healthy living tips

The Kidney Group@thekidneygroup – Consistently voted Top Nephrology Practice in So Florida, we bring you kidney and related health news with commentary by our board certified nephrologists.

World Kidney Day@worldkidneyday – World Kidney Day's objective is to raise awareness globally of the importance of Kidney Health and to increase screening for Chronic Kidney Disease

You can also follow me at **SlowItDownCKD** on Twitter for daily nuggets of CKD information.

Did I miss any? Which do you follow that I haven't listed here? I showed you mine. Now show me yours.

From Nigeria to Neurons

2/25/13   I spent the morning trying to figure out how to call Nigeria. When I started, I had no idea it was a problem. Then Sprint told me international calls are not on my plan. So I turned to the office phone, a landline. Well, Cox apparently doesn't believe in direct dialing to other countries so an operator helped me place the call. The result: a tinny conversation with a friend of the heart who will be attending our wedding as a result of this call.

Of course, that got me to thinking about Nigeria directly. My friend is a retired nurse and told me of having a teaching hospital there decades ago. Aha, time to research.

It looks like Nigeria has its own share of kidney problems. According to one article, The Secretary FCT {Federal Capital Territory in Abuja} Health and Human Services Secretariat – Dr. Demola Onakomaiya – feels that kidney disease is increasing far too rapidly and that the two existing dialysis and intensive care units need to be, and are being, augmented by new hospitals and the expanded services being provided in existing hospitals.

Since Nigeria is home to a whopping 20% of the blacks in the world, this should not be a surprise. I've written repeatedly about the black population having a higher risk and incidence of Chronic Kidney Disease and that no one quite knows why this is.

According to Dr. Ola Akinboboye, Associate Professor of Clinical Medicine at Cornell University, President of the Association of Black Cardiologists, and native Nigerian:

"African Americans are six times more likely than Caucasians to develop hypertension-related kidney failure. I always stress the importance of controlling hypertension to my patients because even mild elevations in blood pressure are associated with significantly high risk of kidney failure particularly in African Americans."

Six times, ladies and gentlemen! Six times. That makes me irrationally fear for every black friend I have.

The American Kidney Fund tells us about the increased risk factors for high blood pressure {hypertension} which is in itself risk causing for Chronic Kidney Disease.

• Are over 45 years of age
• Are overweight
• Are African American
• Have a family member with hypertension
• Are not physically active
• Eat a diet high in salt
• Drink too much alcohol
• Smoke

Notice the third item on the list.

According to Jane Brody's *NY Times* article in January of this year, only 52% of the 76 million hypertension sufferers in this country have their blood pressure under control. She offers these possible reasons.

"About 20 percent of affected adults don't know they have high blood pressure, perhaps because they never or rarely see a doctor who checks their pressure.

Of the 80 percent who are aware of their condition, some don't appreciate how serious it can be and fail to get treated, even when their doctors say they should.

Some who have been treated develop bothersome side effects, causing them to abandon therapy or to use it haphazardly.

Many others do little to change lifestyle factors, like obesity, lack of exercise and a high-salt diet, that can make hypertension harder to control."

She also interviews a physician about specific medications for specific hypertension causes.

I remember well and sadly my mom telling me she wasn't taking her blood pressure medication because she didn't want to be one of those old people who take pills for everything. I am one of those old {er} people who take my hypertension medication… and my cholesterol medication…and my arthritis medication. I see where not taking her pills led and I'm not going down that path.

I wish she had lived to read about this.

"Researchers from Sweden spotted the previously unknown cluster of nerve cells in the brains of mice, finding the cells affected the animals' blood pressure and other cardiovascular functions. If these neurons also exist in human brains, scientists and doctors may have a new avenue for tackling hypertension (chronically high blood pressure) and other heart problems."

Let's not get all excited just yet. First the neurons have to be identified in humans, if they even exist in us. Makes me think of all those who don't comply with their doctor's orders to take medication or are unaware of their own hypertension with new hope.

I've come far afield today: from my wedding, to Nigeria, to blacks' higher risk of CKD due to hypertension, to non-compliance, to possible neuron induced hbp. That is just how my mind works. No wonder Bear has trouble following my discussions sometimes! Poor man.

It Is Not All in Your Mind; It's In Your Organs, Too.

3/4/13   There's so much to share that I wasn't sure what to concentrate on this week... until I spoke with Nima. We went from discussing birthday parties to Bat Mitzvahs to lithium.

According to Wikipedia,

"Trace amounts of lithium are present in all organisms. The element serves no apparent vital biological function, since animals and plants survive in good health without it. Nonvital functions have not been ruled out. The lithium ion Li^+ administered as any of several lithium salts has proved to be useful as a mood-stabilizing drug in the treatment of bipolar disorder, due to neurological effects of the ion in the human body."

The operant word in this definition is SALTS.

There were two Plenary Sessions I attended at the Southwest Nephrology Conference last weekend. It was at the second one, 'Psychiatric issues in kidney patients' that I suddenly sprang to attention. What was this man saying? Something about lithium doubling the risk for Chronic Kidney Disease?

And I was off... how many psychiatric patients knew that fact? How many of their caretakers knew that just in case the patient was not responsible at the time of treatment? What about children? Did their parents know? Was a screening for CKD performed BEFORE lithium was prescribed?

26 million Americans have kidney disease that is not yet diagnosed. What if one of these psychiatric patients belongs to that group? What if they all do? Currently, kidney disease is the ninth leading cause of death in the United States. Ninth!!! Are these undiagnosed psychiatric patients moving it to the eighth? And what about the 73 million at risk for kidney disease due to high blood pressure, diabetes, or family history? Are they being given lithium without screening?

I decided to dig deeper, as I often do. Again and again on different sites about side effects of different psychiatric drugs, I found warnings that patients need to have a complete medical exam before starting the drug and then periodical exams to check whether or not the patient has developed some damage from taking the drug. Here's my question: do these exams include kidney screening?

First I looked at my Twitter feed and found this.

"The $1.6-million federally funded project — First Nations Community Based Screening to Improve Kidney Health and Dialysis — will launch in March.

The project, co-led by Manitoba First Nations' Diabetes Integration Project and Manitoba Health's Manitoba Renal Program, provides early detection and treatment to several First Nations communities.

Detection of the disease in people as young as eight can take less than 15 minutes. The article deals with a KEEP type program {The National Kidney Foundation's Kidney Early Evaluation Program} for some Canadian First Nations and is included here to demonstrate the growing awareness of the need to screen for kidney disease."

Other than that article, there is nothing about screening for kidney disease. If medical practitioners aren't aware of the prevalence of CKD – and, obviously, I am not referring to the entire medical profession – how can psychiatric practitioners be expected to know to do this?

I am not a psychiatric patient so I don't know what the screening process is first hand. However, I do know people who have confided in me that they are taking drugs for some psychiatric condition. Big mouth here always asks what effect that drug might have on their kidneys... or liver for that matter since such drugs may hit the liver negatively.

That is not enough. We need many more big mouths to ask the right question about drugs: How will this affect my kidneys?

I'm asking for one, no two, wedding presents from each and every one of you.
    1.   Have yourself tested for kidney disease
    2.   Before you take any drug for any reason, ask how it will affect your kidneys.

1885... To The Present

3/11/13 1885 is my favorite year. Don't ask me why because I don't know. Maybe it's a reincarnation thing, maybe it's a time travel thing, maybe it's not. All I know is that it draws me like honey draws flies.

So what does this have to do with Chronic Kidney Disease you ask? I know what dresses, shoes, and Western vests looked like in 1885, but not what the face of Chronic Kidney Disease looked like at that time. So I did what I do best: researched. This was one of the few times I didn't succeed. I tried every combination of search parameters I could think of. I finally decided to put a time cap on the research. Nothing, nada.

Then I did one of those mentally smack your forehead thingies. Of course I wasn't finding information about Chronic Kidney Disease at that time. It wasn't as yet recognized as a disease.

According to Dr. G. Eknoyan of Baylor College's Department of Medicine's Renal Section

"Nephrology is a young discipline. Several events contributed to its emergence during the years following World War Two. First was the increasing interest in studies of kidney function and physiology that started as part of the war effort during World War Two and was fostered during the post-war boom by the newly established National Institutes of Health and the flourishing pharmaceutical industry. Second was the introduction in the mid-1900s of new technologies directly relevant to the care of individuals with kidney disease, specifically dialysis and kidney biopsy."

Dr. Eknoyan attributes his information to S.J. Peitzman's book *Dropsy, Dialysis, Transplant, A Short History of Failing Kidneys* published by Johns Hopkins University Press in Baltimore in 2007.

I was astonished to discover that The National Kidney Foundation Kidney Disease Outcomes Quality Initiative (NKF KDOQI ™) was not put into place until 1997 and then updated only five years later in 2002. No wonder I had so much trouble even attempting to discover the face of Chronic Kidney Disease in 1885. I was over a century too early.

There is so much information on their site about CKD in conjunction with diabetes, hypertension, diet, age, treatment, and dyslipidemia {high cholesterol} – to mention just a few of the categories – that I urge you to explore the site yourself.

I was surprised that their chart does not differentiate between stages 3A and 3B, although both are listed. I was just a bit perturbed at one of The Renal Association's statements, although I recognized its validity.

"Most patients with Stage 3 CKD are older, and only a minority go on to get more serious kidney disease."

The older part didn't thrill me, but the "only a minority" part sure did. According to Wikipedia,

"British guidelines distinguish between stage 3A (GFR 45–59) and stage 3B (GFR 30–44) for purposes of screening and referral."

Yet, my nephrologist, who is not British and practices right here in Arizona, is the one who explained to me that I am Stage 3A.

I'm convinced that the renal diet plays a very large part in keeping dialysis at bay. I'm also delighted at how easy it's become to stay within the guidelines of the diet. Last night, we went to a restaurant for dinner. I made exactly two substitutions to the printed menu, skipped dessert and was perfectly within my guidelines as to portion size, vegetable and protein restrictions, and carbohydrate restrictions, too.

While this month is National Kidney Month, did you know that World Kidney Day is this Thursday, March 14th?

To Stress or Not To Stress

3/18/13 The only stress I have is that which I impose upon myself. Stress? Hmmm? What does that do to the kidneys? But wait, maybe it would be more prudent to explore just what stress is first.

According to the Free Online Medical Dictionary,

"Stress is defined as an organism's total response to environmental demands or pressures."

The site goes on to explain the description, causes, symptoms, diagnosis, treatment, alternative treatment, prognosis and prevention of stress. While this was interesting reading, it's not quite germane to the kidneys.

Alright. We have those demands or pressures. But what is our organism's total response? You've got to remember we respond the same way whether the stress is positive or negative.

Ready? First you feel the fight or flight syndrome which means you are releasing hormones. The adrenal glands which secrete these hormones lay right on top of your kidneys. Your blood sugar raises, too, and there's an increase in both heart rate and blood pressure. Diabetes {blood sugar} and hypertension {blood pressure} both play a part in Chronic Kidney Disease.

If you still haven't resolved the stress, additional hormones are secreted for more energy.

Still no resolution? Not good. Years, even weeks, of stress can

"...affect the heart, kidneys {and doesn't affecting the heart also affect the kidneys?}, blood pressure {Uh-oh, that also affects the kidneys.} stomach, muscles and joints."

Thank you to Comprehensive Kidney Facts for this information. For those of you who want more technical explanations, I turned to eHow.

"The combination of vasoconstriction (constriction) of blood vessels by small muscles in their walls. When blood vessels constrict, the flow of blood is restricted and increase in blood volume (because of water retention) raises blood pressure, which can, over time, translate into chronic hypertension {high blood pressure}. Persistent water retention as an outcome of prolonged elevations in stress hormones can also produce edema {swelling}."

Stress management seems to be part of keeping our already compromised kidneys from deteriorating even more. Naturally, the next question should be what IS stress management?

You're already exercising half an hour a day {You are, aren't you?} That's to control your weight, blood pressure, cholesterol and triglyceride levels. To quote from **What Is It and How Did I Get It? Early Stage Chronic Kidney Disease:**

"The greater your triglycerides, the greater the risk of increasing your creatinine."

Creatinine is:

"... a compound released by voluntary muscle contraction. It tells the body to repair itself and grow stronger."

So it's no great surprise that exercise also lowers your blood pressure, even when it's been raised by stress.

Smoking and alcohol - contrary to popular belief - will only increase your stress levels. I'm wondering if we didn't get the notion they would decrease stress from the movies or television.

Drinking water, but keeping within your daily fluid limits {Mine is 64 ounces, which includes any liquid or frozen liquid such as jello}, can also reduce stress as can anything that relaxes you: music, your pet, a warm bath, playing an instrument, etc.

None of This Matters

3/25/13   Household tips I have learned via prepping the house for the wedding.

1. Contact paper works well on bathroom windows for privacy.
2. Adhesive whiteboard paper makes a good privacy screen on the shower door.
3. Trees and bushes cut back due to frost damage do grow back quickly.
4. Things break at the absolutely worst time: dishwasher, solar water heating panel, a/c.
5. None of this matters.

The most important one is #5. We are preparing for one of the most special days for us – our wedding – and we'll be married whether we discovered these things or not.

But I may not have been here for my wedding day if my Chronic Kidney Disease had not been discovered. Once it was, I was given the tools to retard its progression and seemingly reverse it at times.

An even earlier discovery of my CKD would probably have been better. Okay, so I was seeing a Physician's Assistant who wasn't all that astute. The readings were right there in my blood tests almost a year before I changed to a primary care doctor who actually cared. I really liked the P.A. who had been taking care of me, but learned that liking a person doesn't necessarily mean she is a good medical practitioner.

There are so many ifs here. If I had known earlier, could I have made sure my eGFR {estimated glomerular filtration rate} didn't dip as low as it was when I was finally diagnosed? If I had been seeing a doctor rather than a P.A., would she have caught the CKD earlier? If the blood tests had been read carefully, would I have had the opportunity to get to work on preventing rapid progression in the decline of my kidneys?

I will never know the answers to those questions, so – as #5 says – none of this matters ... for me. For you? That's another story.

Have you ever heard of KEEP? That's the Kidney Early Evaluation Program. Notice the word 'Early' in the title. With CKD, the earlier you can detect the disease, the better. According to the National Kidney Foundation,

"The goals of KEEP are to:

- Raise awareness about kidney disease especially among 'high risk' individuals
- Provide free testing for people at increased risk for kidney disease
- Encourage people 'at risk' to visit a clinician and follow the treatment plan recommended
- Provide educational information so that 'at risk' individuals can prevent or delay kidney damage
- Provide clinician referrals for follow-up care, if needed
- Provide ongoing information and support"

The KEEP Program is for all people, but the 'high risk' ones are the ones that may need to take immediate action. What is 'high risk' you ask? According to The National Kidney Center these are the high risk people:

"High risk groups for Chronic Kidney Disease (CKD) include those with diabetes, hypertension and a family history of kidney disease. African Americans, Hispanics, Pacific Islanders, Native Americans and Seniors are also at increased risk."

That definition covers quite a bit of ground. For example, I have hypertension {high blood pressure} and am a senior. I don't know if there's any history of kidney disease in my family since the cousins my age don't know of any, but our parents would never discuss their health with us.

Alright, so we need early detection. Now, where can you find that? On the homepage of The National Kidney Foundation, there is an orange bar running across the page. It has different tabs on it. Hit the one that reads "Events." Once you get to that page, scroll down and you'll see the words, "Find a KEEP Screening Near You." Hit it. Voila! You've found your local KEEP Screening.

The logical question here is, "What if there isn't one near me?" You don't have to travel across state lines to find out if you have CKD. Speak with your PCP {primary care doctor} and ask him or her to run a blood test and a urine test. While the results may not be crystal clear to a doctor who is not a nephrologist {kidney and hypertension specialist}, high or low readings will be marked. They will let your PCP know there may be a kidney function problem.

The National Kidney Disease Education Program at The U.S. Department of Health and Human Services provides the following information.

1. A blood test checks your GFR, which tells how well your kidneys are filtering. GFR stands for glomerular filtration rate.
2. A urine test checks for albumin. Albumin is a protein that can pass into the urine when the kidneys are damaged.

If necessary, meaning if your kidney function is compromised, your PCP will make certain you get to a nephrologist promptly. This specialist will conduct more intensive tests that include:

Blood:

BUN – BUN stands for blood urea nitrogen.

Creatinine - The creatinine blood test measures the level of creatinine in the blood. This test is done to see how well your kidneys work.

Urine:
Creatinine clearance - The creatinine clearance test helps provide information about how well the kidneys are working. The test compares the creatinine level in urine with the creatinine level in blood.

Timidly Exploring Dialysis

4/1/13   While I've only gained a few pounds {no, really}, my body has finally decided to show my age. Out went the tightly fitted dressy T-shirts that accentuated the belly. Out went the fancy blouses with no room for the droopy bust. Out went the casual dress pants with their tight waistlines. Out went the maxi skirts that now reached the floor since I've shrunk.

And it struck me. I looked something like the peritoneal dialysis patient Walter A. Hunt mentions in his book *Kidney Disease: A Guide for Living.*

"Peritoneal dialysis also causes weight gain and an increased waistline, which are mostly caused by fluid retention. It may be difficult to find clothes that fit properly, because your abdomen may become quite large."

I began to wonder what else I don't know about either of these medical procedures and ended up where I almost always do: MedlinePlus, a service of U.S. National Library of Medicine and National Institutes of Health. This is what I found there.

"When your kidneys are healthy, they clean your blood. They also make hormones that keep your bones strong and your blood healthy. When your kidneys fail, you need treatment to replace the work your kidneys used to do. Unless you have a kidney transplant, you will need a treatment called dialysis.

There are two main types of dialysis: hemodialysis and peritoneal dialysis. Both types filter your blood to rid your body of harmful wastes, extra salt and water. Hemodialysis does that with a machine. Peritoneal dialysis uses the lining of your abdomen, called the peritoneal membrane, to filter your blood. Each type has both risks and benefits. They also require that you follow a special diet. Your doctor can help you decide the best type of dialysis for you."

This may be old news to those of you who are already dealing with renal dialysis and it was to me, too, but what about those people who are still in early stage or who love someone in early stage? They don't need to be bewildered when {if} this becomes necessary for them down the road, the way they were when they were first diagnosed with Chronic Kidney Disease.

As much as I deplore the thought of dialysis – I can't stand anyone fiddling with me, not even for a manicure or a massage – this may become a necessity somewhere down the line for me – or you. We all know I intend to be one of the 80% of CKD patients who never progress beyond stage 3… but what if I'm not? What if you're not?

Peeking At Transplantation

4/8/13   I am not morbid; I'm just plain realistic. And that's why we'll take a little peek at transplantation today. Remember that I'm not a doctor and I didn't want to know anything about this ever. But it is a fact in some lives. Sure I don't want to have one of those lives and I'm doing everything I can to avoid it, yet….

Do you know about the *Transplant Community Outreach* page on Facebook? They asked me to be their kidney 'expert' right after **What Is It and How Did I Get It? Early Stage Chronic Kidney Disease** was published. I balked since I certainly didn't feel like an expert and knew nothing about transplantation. The administrators went back and forth with me until I understood they didn't expect me to know everything, just to remind the transplantees what it had been like in the early stages and keep them informed about what new discoveries have been made since their own time in the early stages of Chronic Kidney Disease. I was comfortable doing that.

You already know that when your kidney function decreases to 10 or 15%, depending upon your nephrologist's views, you need outside help. By this I mean, from outside your body. We timidly explored dialysis last week. A word about that. There is so much more that I've learned about dialysis while I was researching for that blog. If you'd also like to learn more – whether you're at the point of needing it or not – I urge you to do more research on your own.

Or, if you're not comfortable researching, go to one of the national kidney organizations. They will give you clear, simply stated explanations with diagrams and will list other sources. I would start with Medlineplus, a service of The National Institute of Diabetes and Digestive and Kidney. That is where this definition of a kidney transplant is from.

"A kidney transplant is an operation that places a healthy kidney in your body. The transplanted kidney takes over the work of the two kidneys that failed, so you no longer need dialysis.

During a transplant, the surgeon places the new kidney in your lower abdomen and connects the artery and vein of the new kidney to your artery and vein. Often, the new kidney will start making urine as soon as your blood starts flowing through it. But sometimes it takes a few weeks to start working.

Many transplanted kidneys come from donors who have died. Some come from a living family member. The wait for a new kidney can be long.

If you have a transplant, you must take drugs for the rest of your life, to keep your body from rejecting the new kidney."

I find people cringe at the thought of taking drugs for that long, but think of the alternative... or lack of one. There is quite a bit of information packed into that concise definition.

A couple of reminders taken from the glossary of **What Is It and How Did I Get It? Early Stage Chronic Kidney Disease**.

1. Arteries are the vessels that carry blood *from* the heart.

2. Veins are the vessels that carry blood *toward* the heart.

In the last decade, there has been experimentation with taking the donor kidney laparoscopically. That means using extremely small instruments which require extremely small incisions into the abdomen of the donor. I haven't seen any articles that are negative about this and it cuts down on the recovery time for the live donor. Since we each have two kidneys and it is possible to live with one, someone who matches may donate a kidney to you. Otherwise, you will receive something called a cadaver kidney, meaning one which comes from someone who has just died.

Recently, according to ScienceBlog, this marvelous procedure of removing donor kidneys laparoscopically has been further improved by using only one incision in the belly button which is lost within the navel folds once it is healed. The idea is to make it more comfortable for the living donor so that more living donors can be found.

As for the person receiving the kidney, you will be on anti-rejection drugs for the rest of your life. Your body is designed to reject foreign bodies – including organs. You'll also need to pay attention to exercise, diet, sleep, and stress sort of like with CKD.

Some people choose not to take on that challenge. It was only through my buddy's death that I came to realize not everyone wants to prolong their life if it means doing what they don't feel they can.

Weight a Minute

4/15/13 Keeping your weight down is one of the ways to help retard the progression of the disease. How? By not allowing yourself to become obese. Obviously, if you keep gaining weight, you can become obese. Obesity is one of the contributing factors for developing diabetes. Diabetes may lead to, and complicates, the treatment of, CKD. Based on my BMI {Body Mass Index} I am obese. This is from ***What Is It and How Did I Get It? Early Stage Chronic Kidney Disease***.

"The BMI formula was something about your weight divided by the sum of your height in inches squared times 703. I think. I have researched and researched this, but still do not understand it. I did discover later on that there are free BMI Calculators online, …, so you really only need to know your height and weight."

Medical News Today published this information in an article:

"A University of Bristol team, with funding from the British Heart Foundation (BHF), has now identified that a target found to be critical in the brain's regulation of body weight, is also crucially involved in the development of obesity-associated conditions. Researchers describe the mechanism behind a key molecule, known as melanocortin-4-receptor (MC4R), whose mutation or loss in both human and animal models has shown to cause severe obesity with type 2 diabetes."

The title of the article is *Scientists Identify Culprit In Obesity-Associated High Blood Pressure*. Hmmm, high blood pressure {hypertension}, another contributor to CKD. This is preliminary research so we can't just pop a pill that will magically control our weight. We need to do that ourselves.

If you read a different article from News Health, you'll find that obesity also may lead to a drop in vitamin D, something we can't afford as CKD patients. This is the vitamin that regulates calcium and phosphorous blood levels as well as promoting bone formation, among other tasks. It also affects the immune system. If you're like me at stage 3A, you're already taking vitamin D supplements since we need to control phosphorous levels, which means we cannot afford to lose any more of it.

Yet another caution about obesity from Medical News Today is not only for CKD patients but any woman of child bearing age. The headline says it all: *Obese Women Taking Certain Contraceptive May Be At Increased Risk For Type 2 Diabetes*. Keep in mind that diabetes, as mentioned before, may contribute to the development of CKD.

According to DaVita:

- … people with a BMI 35 or greater had higher death rates than normal weight, overweight and mildly obese patients, so becoming more obese is a concern.
- Obese people are more likely to have chronic diseases like diabetes, high blood pressure and heart disease, which could mean they receive more medical care and monitoring compared to normal weight people.
- Excess weight may be a source of energy during illness or injury—a benefit the lean person does not have.
- A person can have different degrees of health and fitness regardless of their BMI or weight. Factors such as nutrition status, diseases, health history, where fat is stored (abdominal vs. lower body), exercise and eating habits influence your level of fitness.

The message here is that while excess weight may not affect your general health and may even be of some benefit during times of ill health, we have a chronic disease and cannot afford the luxury of the benefits in being overweight.

Guilty Pleasures

4/22/13   I read this phrase somewhere and that's what today blog is: my guilty pleasure. It's my pleasure because my mission is to keep informing about Chronic Kidney Disease and it's my guilt because I indulge myself in using my own life experiences to ease into this information.

So let's get to the heart of today's blog: pregnancy when you have Chronic Kidney Disease. According to the physicians' journal **_BMJ_**:

"Pregnant women with chronic renal {kidney} disease adapt poorly to a gestational {pregnancy} increase in renal blood flow. This may accelerate their decline in renal function and lead to a poor pregnancy outcome."

That blatantly gives you the bad news first, but it's not the end of any thought of pregnancy with CKD. The following is a 1980 view of pregnancy's effect on kidney disease from Webdoc. Keep that date in mind since it is 33 years ago.

- Increase in proteinuria {protein in the urine}
- risk of preeclampsia {hypertension -a sharp rise in blood pressure, albuminuria - leakage of large amounts of the protein albumin into the urine, and edema – swelling of the hands, feet, and face}
- worsening of anemia {low red blood cell level}
- lessening of renal function.

While I've paraphrased, it's clear pregnancy with CKD was frowned upon all those years ago.

Okay, lots of definitions in the above outdated article. Let's see what thoughts about the subject are fairly current.

Pregnancy and Chronic Kidney Disease: A Challenge in All CKD Stages is the the title of an article I found on the site of _The Clinical Journal of the American Society of Nephrology_.

The word 'challenge' caught my eye, so I did my best to understand the article which summarized information garnered between 2000 and 2009 about the subject. According to the article, more cases of CKD were discovered during pregnancy than had been expected.

"Chronic Kidney Disease complicates an increasing number of pregnancies, and at least 4% of childbearing-aged women are afflicted by this condition. Although diabetic nephropathy {kidney disease from long term diabetes.} is the most common type of Chronic Kidney Disease found in pregnant women, a variety of other primary and systemic kidney diseases also commonly occur. In the setting of mild maternal primary Chronic Kidney Disease (serum creatinine <1.3 mg/dL) without poorly controlled hypertension, most pregnancies result in live births and maternal kidney function is unaffected. In cases of more moderate and severe maternal primary Chronic Kidney Disease, the incidence of fetal prematurity, low birth weight, and death increase substantially, and the risk of accelerated irreversible decline in maternal kidney function, proteinuria, and hypertensive complications rise dramatically.

In addition to kidney function, maternal hypertension and proteinuria portend negative outcomes and are important factors to consider when risk stratifying for fetal and maternal complications. In the setting of diabetic nephropathy and lupus nephropathy {kidney inflammation caused by lupus}, other systemic disease features such as disease activity, the presence of antiphospholipid antibodies {antibodies that might be in your blood and might increase the incidence of blood clotting and pregnancy termination}, and glycemic control {eating low carbohydrate foods to help manage diabetes} play important roles in determining pregnancy outcomes. Concomitant with advances in obstetrical management and kidney disease treatments, it appears that the historically dismal maternal and fetal outcomes have greatly improved."

The above is taken from *Chronic Kidney Disease and Pregnancy: Maternal and Fetal Outcomes* by Michael J. Fischer, which is dated April, 2007. I included the entire paragraph since it makes so clear that pregnancy outcomes "have greatly improved." And that was six years ago!

I seem to be having trouble finding anything more recent, so I'll summarize what I have found.

1. Speak with your nephrologist about a high risk team before you become pregnant, if possible.
2. Pregnancy in early stages of CKD has better outcomes.
3. CKD may be discovered during pregnancy.
4. Pregnancy is not an impossibility if you have CKD.
5. Treatment in pregnancy in CKD is continually improving.
6. The risks are caused by increased renal blood flow along with other factors.

Don't let CKD cause you to miss out on one of the wonders of life, but don't be foolish. Take care of that baby you intend to bring into the world by taking care of its mother.

Reminder: giving birth to a baby is not the only way to become a mother.

The Wild West Isn't So Wild These Days

4/29/13   Native Americans have the highest rate of diabetes in the world, yet they comprise only 1.5% of this country's population. This is striking when you think about it.

While Caucasians are usually diagnosed around age 60, Native Americans develop diabetes most often in their mid-thirties. All those extra years to be at a substantial risk of CKD!

According to DaVita,

"The rate of end stage renal disease among Native Americans with diabetes is six times higher than among non-Native Americans."

You can read more about Native Americans, diabetes, and Chronic Kidney Disease on DaVita's website.

Already underfunded, the Indian Health Service – which, by the way, is a division of The United States Department of Health and Human Services – has been hit hard this year by budget cuts. So we have budget cuts to an already underfunded program.

Arizona is a fairly large state with over 6% of the population being Native American. There are 21 federally recognized tribes here with two others petitioning for recognition as of March, 2007. According to Native American Tribes by State, these are the federally recognized tribes as of that same date.

- Ak Chin Indian Community of the Maricopa (Ak Chin) Indian Reservation
- Cocopah Tribe of Arizona
- Colorado River Indian Tribes of the Colorado River Indian Reservation (Arizona and California)
- Fort McDowell Yavapai Nation
- Fort Mojave Indian Tribe (Arizona, California and Nevada)
- Gila River Indian Community of the Gila River Indian Reservation
- Havasupai Tribe of the Havasupai Reservation
- Hopi Tribe of Arizona

- Hualapai Indian Tribe of the Hualapai Indian Tribe Reservation
- Kaibab Band of Paiute Indians of the Kaibab Indian Reservation
- Navajo Nation (Arizona, New Mexico and Utah)
- Pascua Yaqui Tribe of Arizona
- Quechan Tribe of the Fort Yuma Indian Reservation (Arizona and California)
- Salt River Pima-Maricopa Indian Community of the Salt River Reservation
- San Carlos Apache Tribe of the San Carlos Reservation
- San Juan Southern Paiute Tribe of Arizona
- Tohono O'odham Nation of Arizona (formerly the Papago)
- Tonto Apache Tribe of Arizona
- White Mountain Apache Tribe of the Fort Apache Reservation
- Yavapai-Apache Nation of the Camp Verde Indian Reservation
- Yavapai-Prescott Tribe of the Yavapai Reservation

The Less Than Sexy Sinuses

5/6/13   I have a whopping sinus infection, a bacterial, non-contagious infection.

Viral commonly means an airborne virus which doesn't respond to drugs since it needs a host to live in, and so, is already inside our cells by the time we become ill. One way we spread this type of infection is by sneezing and coughing in public.

Bacteria, on the other hand, do respond to drugs like the 500 mg. of ciprofloxacin I'm taking twice a day for ten days. I ran this prescription from my primary care doctor by both the pharmacist and the nephrologist to make certain the drug wouldn't harm my kidneys… and I trust my primary care doctor! Bacteria need no host and are cells in their own right.

The obvious question is, "How did I suddenly develop an infection in this part of the body of all places?" According to MedlinePlus,

'Sinusitis can be acute, lasting for less than four weeks, or chronic, lasting much longer. Acute sinusitis often starts as a cold, which then turns into a bacterial infection. Allergies, pollutants, nasal problems and certain diseases can also cause sinusitis."

Well, I have allergies. And sinusitis just means an inflammation of the sinuses – which is what an infection is.

But what, if anything, does this have to do with Chronic Kidney Disease? You've got to remember that your immune system is already compromised. Your kidneys aren't working at 100% {See your GFR.}. Your medications have to be monitored and sometimes modified. If your body is not releasing the meds at full capacity via the kidneys that aren't working at full capacity, you may need to take less of them, lower the strength, or lengthen the time between doses.

Back to the sinuses. I knew where they were because I could feel them when I first realized I was ill. I'm still not that quick to realize when I'm ill and was at my primary care doctor's office for the required annual Medicare Wellness visit {How's that for irony?} when she quickly changed it to a non-Wellness visit and asked me to schedule another Wellness visit.

The Mayo Clinic has this to say about acute sinusitis:

"Acute sinusitis (acute rhinosinusitis) causes the cavities around your nasal passages (sinuses) to become inflamed and swollen. This interferes with drainage and causes mucus to build up.

With acute sinusitis, it may be difficult to breathe through your nose. The area around your eyes and face may feel swollen, and you may have throbbing facial pain or a headache."

Before we get any more detailed here, a few reminders are in order {taken from *What Is It and How Did I Get It? Early Stage Chronic Kidney Disease*'s Glossary}.

Acute – Extremely painful, severe or serious, quick onset, of short duration; the opposite of chronic.

Antibiotic – Medication used to treat infection.

Chronic – Long term, the opposite of acute.

Chronic Kidney Disease – Damage to the kidneys for more than three months, which cannot be reversed but may be slowed.

GFR – Glomerular filtration rate which determines both the stage of kidney disease and how well the kidneys are functioning.

Medicare – U.S. government health insurance for those over 65, those having certain special needs, or those who have end stage renal disease.

Nephrologist – Renal or kidney and hypertension specialist.

I tend to have the acute kind of sinus infection. I can't see making this a lifelong practice, so I'll try to avoid it. I'm not quite sure how just yet. Here are some suggestions I found at essortment.com which calls itself "your source for knowledge." I am not familiar with the site, although I did like that they differentiate between viral and bacterial sinusitis.

"Be sure to blow your nose frequently to prevent a mucous buildup. Apply a warm, but not hot, washcloth or compress to your face for five or ten minutes at a time, perhaps twice a day, to help loosen stuffy passages. Very warm showers or baths likewise can help to release tight muscles and open the sinuses to let them flow. Enjoy hot tea on a regular basis. Filled with flavonoids and antioxidants that can track down and kill bacteria, tea's steam can open up and loosen your sinus passages to prevent problems from developing."

I felt as if I had swollen glands, could barely talk, could not stop blowing my nose, and {the worst part for a CKD patient who avoids NSAIDS} had a headache that stopped me cold.

Eat and Be Well

5/13/13   Today's blog is going to be about food. Keeping that in mind, I found this general guideline to healthy eating on so many different diabetes sites that it would be unfair to cite just one.

The Basics

Your body needs the right vitamins, minerals, and other nutrients to stay healthy. A healthy diet means that you are eating:

- Vegetables, fruits, whole grains, and fat-free or low-fat milk products
- Seafood, poultry, lean meats, eggs, beans, peas, seeds, and nuts

Limit foods high in:

- Cholesterol, sodium (salt), and added sugars
- *Trans* fats – *Trans* fats may be in foods like cakes, cookies, stick margarines, and fried foods.
- Saturated fats – These fats come from animal products like cheese, fatty meats, whole milk, and butter.
- Refined grains – Food products with refined grains include white bread, noodles, white rice, and flour tortillas

What I found interesting here is that what the general population is urged to eat is not that much different than what we early stage Chronic Kidney Disease patients are told to eat. We do have to limit the fruits and vegetables to three different sized portions of each. The portion depends on the particular fruit or vegetable. We also need to cap our limited types of seafood, poultry, lean meats, and eggs to five ounces per day. As for seeds and nuts, those are no-no's for us.

Look at the foods we should avoid. Look familiar? Take a look at the renal diet your nutritionist gave you and you'll find them on that as foods to limit - or avoid, too.

The previous information was taken from websites dealing with diabetes because this is the leading cause of Chronic Kidney Disease and vice-versa. That's another reason to watch your intake of foods with a high glycemic index – the indicator of how quickly your blood sugar rises after eating the food – which includes not only what we usually consider sweets, but ice cream, too.

You know we need to stay as healthy as possible, including keeping our weight down. One way to do that is NOT skipping breakfast. Why? This is how study researcher Dr. Tony Goldstone, M.D., Ph.D. of Imperial College London in the UK explains it.

"Through both the participants' MRI results and observations of how much they ate at lunch, we found ample evidence that fasting made people hungrier, and increased the appeal of high-calorie foods and the amount people ate."

You can read more about the study that led him to come to this conclusion on Medical News Today {MNT}.

You need to understand that skipping breakfast {literally breaking the fast you incur while you sleep} is a form of fasting. If you take medication that requires food along with it, you're also delaying the effects of the medication since you're not taking it until later in the day.

Here's an interesting finding on a study published in *The Journal of Renal Nutrition* in 2009.

"Long-term fish consumption was independently associated with improved kidney function among elderly individuals, a finding that extends the current knowledge regarding the benefits of fish intake on human health."

But we knew that, didn't we?

By the way, are you taking Omega 3 {Fish oil} supplements? There's a theory it helps retard the progress of CKD. I've been taking it all five years since my diagnosis and I'm still at stage 3A.

While that's something I would suggest {Please remember: I'm not a doctor.} you need to run my suggestions by your nephrologist before you even think of acting on them!

Something I will caution you about is grapefruit or grapefruit juice. The following is from HealthDay.

"Even small amounts of grapefruit or grapefruit juice have the potential to cause sudden death, acute kidney failure, respiratory failure, gastrointestinal bleeding and other serious side effects when paired with these medications."

And star fruit {Carambola}. Avoid it at ALL costs, because the cost could be your life. It is toxic to people with Chronic Kidney Disease. It's a tropical fruit so chances are you're not going to run into it too often. I am so glad I wasn't adventurous enough to try it in Nigeria all those years ago.

I took the following quote from an article beguilingly entitled *It's not just what you eat, but when you eat it.*

"When a species' typical daily rhythm is thrown off, changes in metabolism also happen. For example, in people, night shift workers have an increased prevalence of obesity and metabolic syndrome, and patients with sleep disorders have a higher risk for developing obesity. Also, less sleep means more weight gain in healthy men and women."

Audrey Hepburn: "Nothing is impossible, the word itself says 'I'm possible'!"

5/20/13   Yes, DaVita IS a dialysis provider, but also invested in the humanity of staving off dialysis as long as possible. On their homepage you can find education about both early and late stage CKD, and dialysis, as well as information on just what CKD is and help in locating a doctor.

This is how I described this company in ***What Is It and How Did I Get It? Early Stage Chronic Kidney Disease***.

"I'd been told about **DaVita** at my doctor's office. This was a website from a private company that provided both the much dreaded dialysis and the much needed kidney education. Maybe that wouldn't be so foreboding for me. I went to the website and clicked on every possible thing I could click on. This was a little better, but it was a dot com – a for profit site. Maybe it was one that offered all this information so that when you needed dialysis, you would turn to them since they had been so helpful all along. And what, if anything, was wrong with that?"

Locally, people have been searching for live support groups and coming up empty. You know you can find the online support groups in the blogroll, but sometimes people want the live interaction.

I clearly remember how frightened I was when I was first diagnosed and thought it meant I was either immediately going to be tethered to a dialysis machine for the rest of my life or die. That fear is simply no longer necessary in this world.

Stop It Before It Starts

5/27/13   There was a question on *SlowItDownCKD***'s Facebook page** about the inoculations that are suggested for those who have Chronic Kidney Disease.

Before we even get to the different kinds of inoculations, why do we need any in the first place? According to DaVita:

"Immunizations may prevent people from contracting other diseases, infections and viruses. The immune system of a person with Chronic Kidney Disease (CKD) becomes weakened, making it difficult to fight off many diseases and infections. Patients with CKD may become more susceptible to illness and even death if they do not receive regular immunization treatment. Getting the proper immunizations is an essential part of a person's kidney care."

I have been on bed rest for several days, ever since I showed up at my primary care physician's office for my Hepatitis B vaccine and was told I'd have to come back for that at a later date. I either had pneumonia or bronchitis. I didn't know. I thought I'd just been pushing my physical limits and needed to take some time off. Why mention that here? Consider it proof that our immune systems become weaker with CKD.

I clearly remember only a few years ago becoming sick for only a day at a time. Then I noticed that maybe once a year I'd end up with the flu which had me down for about ten days. This year, it's been ten days with the flu, ten days with sinusitis, and now whatever this is. Now that I've convinced you they're necessary, what are the inoculations? There are three that DaVita suggests. The first, as mentioned, is Hepatitis-B. Let's go back a little bit and define the disease.

"Hepatitis B is a serious liver infection caused by the hepatitis B virus (HBV). For some people, hepatitis B infection becomes chronic, leading to liver failure, liver cancer or cirrhosis — a condition that causes permanent scarring of the liver."

That's what The Mayo Clinic has to say about it.

"A Hepatitis B infection may lead to kidney failure. What's worse is that some adults never exhibit the symptoms of this disease. Your kidneys are already compromised, as is your immune system. To the best of my knowledge, the drugs to treat Hepatitis B may also adversely affect the kidneys."

Think about it: your liver and your kidneys are the two most important blood filters you have. We already know we need to maintain as steady a blood pressure in the kidneys as we can to do no more damage to them. The liver does this by releasing angiotensin which constricts your blood vessels. Don't forget the liver helps maintain your blood sugars. If it can't do that due to infection, kidney function can be further reduced. The liver also filters toxins and drugs from the blood.

The liver performs quite a few of the metabolic functions necessary to keep you alive, much less healthy, certain of which affect the kidneys. Metabolic means the

"chemical processes occurring within a living cell or organism that are necessary for the maintenance of life,"

according to the dictionary. If your kidneys are already compromised and then your liver is, what happens to your blood pressure and blood sugars without any kind of regulation?

As I researched, I discovered that the liver also converts blood ammonia – which is toxic – into urea. Remember the kidneys turn urea into urine and that the amount of urea directly affects our kidney function. What I didn't know is that Hepatitis B is one of the infections that can inflame the glomeruli. These are the parts of the kidneys that do the filtering.

I'm sure you've all heard of cirrhosis of the liver. Guess what. It can lead to kidney failure. Get the vaccine!

I've spent most of the blog on the Hepatitis B vaccination because it's relatively new and I, for one, didn't know much about it. I've already written several blogs about the flu vaccine, so I'll just add this tidbit from the website of the Southeastern Kidney Council, Inc.

- Cardiovascular disease is the leading cause of death among patients with CKD
- Infectious diseases are the second most common cause of death among cause of death among patients with CKD
- That statement speaks for itself.

Ah, now the third vaccination: Pneumococcal. Sounds terrible, but it's really just the pneumonia inoculation. MedicineNet tells us this is

"a method of preventing a specific type of lung infection (pneumonia) that is caused by pneumococcus bacterium. There are more than 80 different types of pneumococcus bacteria — 23 of them covered by the vaccine. The vaccine is injected into the body to stimulate the normal immune system to produce antibodies that are directed against pneumococcus bacteria."

Naturally, the next question is why CKD patients? Dr. Joseph A. Vassalotti, Chief Medical Officer of the National Kidney Foundation and Dr. William Schaffner, President of the National Foundation for Infectious Diseases have explained it better than I ever could.

"One reason people with CKD are at greater risk for pneumococcal disease is because kidney disease can weaken the immune system and make the body more susceptible to infection.

2. Doctors and researchers have found that infections in people with CKD such as those caused by pneumococcal disease are worse and can be more serious than in people who don't have CKD.

3. In some people, infection can cause death."

Coffee, the Elixir of the Gods (Or Did I Just Make That Up?)

6/4/13 With all that's going on in my life and in the world, I awoke today thinking, "Coffee, today's blog is going to be about coffee!" Of course, as Chronic Kidney Disease patients, we can't run wild in our pursuit of the perfect cup of coffee and how often we can have it. It's 16 ounces {two cups} maximum for me so I want to have the best taste I can.

But it's become one of those once-in-a-while-heaven-descends treats for me. I haven't quite figured out how it can have the "richest, sweetest essence of the darkest tropical island rum" without containing alcohol, despite what it says on the package. That's a topic for another blog. Going a step further in my coffee research, I found an article at Medical News Today that explains the benefits of Greek coffee and how that works. The part that intrigued me was this.

"The endothelium is a layer of cells that lines the blood vessels, which is impacted by lifestyle habits and aging. The researchers focused on coffee because earlier research has proven that moderate coffee intake may decrease the risk of coronary heart disease, they wondered whether it could have a positive impact on other areas of endothelial health."

According to the article based on the findings which were published in *Vascular Journal* earlier this year, it did.

Another article, this one from *Digestive Disease Week,* offered more good news about coffee.

"Coffee consumption helped protect against the autoimmune liver disease known as primary sclerosing cholangitis (PSC), a disorder of the bile ducts that causes inflammation and obstruction and that can lead to transplantation or death."

Coffee does initially raise blood pressure, but it also has the potential to lower it long term... one of life's little dichotomies. Among the other drawbacks of my favorite beverage are the obvious ones: it can contribute to anxiety, insomnia and tremors. Coffee can exacerbate withdrawal symptoms and there is the potential for it increasing the risk of glaucoma.

The article I liked the best during my research is from NBC News. It offered a detailed explanation of how dopamine is elevated by drinking coffee. In layman's terms, that means coffee can make you feel good. As a non-drinker, non-smoker, I can personally attest to the fact that my two cups of coffee per day make me feel great... and not simply in terms of energy.

Keep That Liver Lively

6/10/13 It feels so good to be relatively healthy again. I've spent the last several weeks being tested, running to doctors, and feeling like I just plain didn't want to move… not even for a good cup of coffee. I like the way I feel now. Maybe I rest more than I've been used to, but I get to do whatever I want again. That's the way to live. I like it so much that I intend to keep my life this way.

And that's why I'm taking the series of Hepatitis B inoculations that are recommended for anyone with a compromised immune system. Chronic Kidney Disease presents us with one of those.

According to MedlinePlus, a service of the U.S. National Library of Medicine, National Institutes of Health,

"Hepatitis B is one type of hepatitis – a liver disease – caused by the hepatitis B virus (HBV). Hepatitis B spreads by contact with an infected person's blood, semen or other body fluid. An infected woman can give hepatitis B to her baby at birth."

Let's backtrack for a little etymology here. The Online Etymology Dictionary shows the following.

hepatitis (n.) 1727, coined from Greek *hepatos*, genitive of *hepar* "liver," from PIE root **yekwr-* (cf. Sanskrit*yakrt*, Avestan *yakar*, Persian *jigar*, Latin *jecur*, Old Lithuanian*jeknos* "liver") + *-itis* "inflammation".

While this is probably too much information, we can see that the term comes from the Greek for liver and the Latin for inflammation, and was first commonly used in 1727. The key word here? Liver.

Okay then, what's the big deal with the liver you're probably asking. While it performs over 500 different functions to keep your body going, one of its primary functions is to filter your blood – just like your kidneys. If your kidney function is already compromised, you've got to be careful not to let your liver function become compromised, too.

We've all heard the stories about people with an alcohol dependency dying of cirrhosis – permanent scarring of the liver, but you can have liver damage from any number of causes. Hepatitis B is one of them.

"Hepatitis B is a serious liver infection caused by the hepatitis B virus (HBV). For some people, hepatitis B infection becomes chronic, leading to liver failure, liver cancer or cirrhosis — a condition that causes permanent scarring of the liver. "

That's from The Mayo Clinic. I especially recommend their site because it is written in the English we all know and is easily understood.

According to the handout from the U.S. Department of Health and Human Services' Center for Disease Control and Prevention which I was given by my doctor's medical assistant, the inoculations come in sets of three. I've had the first and was told to come back in a month for the second, with the third scheduled for a month after the second. In other words, they are spaced over a period of three months.

But what if my primary care doctor hadn't recommended these to me, how would I know if I have Hepatitis B? According to MedicineNet:

"Acute hepatitis B is the period of illness that occurs during the first one to four months after acquiring the virus. Only 30% to 50% of adults develop significant symptoms during acute infection. Early symptoms may be non-specific, including fever, a flu-like illness, and joint pains. Symptoms of acute hepatitis may include:

- fatigue,
- loss of appetite,
- nausea,
- jaundice (yellowing of the skin and eyes), and
- pain in the upper right abdomen (due to the inflamed liver)."

Those are fairly common symptoms for many illnesses and as many as half the people with this virus may not know they have it. I might have been one of that 50%. So might you.

For chronic {Long term} Hepatitis B, as with Chronic Kidney Disease, there are no symptoms until the damage is done and the liver starts to fail.

Father's Day Equality Questions

6/17/13 In an abortive attempt to clean off my desk this morning, I came across the March issue *of Nephrology News & Issues* that I'd picked up at the last renal conference I attended. Being a firm believer in multitasking – after all, I was doing the laundry and overseeing the yard maintenance at the same time I was cleaning my desk – I decided to flip through it while I waited for a call from The National Institute of Health. Right there on page 20, I found the following sentence.

"However, both sexes experienced increased risks of all-cause mortality, cardiovascular mortality and ESRD with lower estimated glomerular filtration rate and higher albuminuria."

Let's backtrack a little. Mortality deals with death, cardiovascular mortality with death from diseases of the heart and blood vessels including those in the kidneys; ESRD is End Stage Renal Disease; glomerular filtration rate and albuminuria are used to judge the degree of kidney function decrease.

There was only one thing wrong with this statement of equality as I saw it. What did that "However" deal with? I looked further back in the paragraph and found that a study had been performed at the Johns Hopkins Bloomberg School of Public Health and the Chronic Kidney Disease Prognosis Consortium which found that,

"... the overall risks of all-cause mortality were higher in men at all levels of kidney function."

I finally figured out that men were at higher risk of any medical cause of death whether they had kidney disease or not, while women had heightened mortality only if they had kidney disease. So, men and women aren't equal?

My research sensors started tingling. What else was different about men and women with Chronic Kidney Disease?

According to a study published in US National Library of Medicine:

"This exploratory analysis of the MDRD study indicates a slower mean GFR decline in women as compared with men. The slower mean GFR decline and suggestive evidence of a lesser beneficial effect of the low protein diet and low blood pressure interventions in women suggest that gender differences should be considered in trials of the effects of these interventions on the progression of renal disease."

This is an older study published in 1998 and deals with gender differences in trials. MDRD means modification of diet in renal disease. So, the study deals with whatever gender differences are associated with adhering to the renal diet.

The 2007 article by Qiu-Li Zhang[*] and Dietrich Rothenbacher concludes with the following sentence.

"Accurately detecting CKD in special groups remains inadequate, particularly among elderly persons, females or other ethnic groups such as Asians."

So first, it is suggested that women be included in CKD trials; then we're told it's difficult to get information about women with CKD.

Aha! An article about a current study from the same Johns Hopkins Bloomberg School of Public Health and the Chronic Kidney Disease Prognosis Consortium (CKD-PC) mentioned above is posted at Science Daily. It establishes that men and women are equal as far as Chronic Kidney Disease.

"Our results contrast with some previous studies suggesting that the association of estimated glomerular filtration rate with mortality is weaker in women. We found the association between Chronic Kidney Disease and mortality risk to be as strong in women as in men. Low estimated glomerular filtration rate or albuminuria should be considered at least as potent a risk factor in women as it is in men," said Josef Coresh, MD, PhD, MHS, the Consortium's principal investigator and professor in the Bloomberg School's Department of Epidemiology.

It Isn't What I Thought It Would Be

6/24/13   I had my blog for today mentally written before I even sat down at the computer tonight. I met with Dr. Jennifer Weil, of The Phoenix Epidemiology and Clinical Research Branch {PECRB} of the National Institutes of Health {NIH} Research Clinic on Saturday. Although a research nephrologist {Specialist in the kidneys and high blood pressure}, she is highly involved in Chronic Kidney Disease education and prevention. She's so involved that she's actually written material that had wonderfully apt analogies of her own devising. Those were what I had planned to write about today.

On Saturday, Dr. Weil gave me a DVD of her informational slide show and permission to use any or all of it for my own devices... or so we thought. Once I sat down to write the blog and choose the slides I was going to use, I discovered she'd given me a DVD of another project, *Looking Out for Our Health – Slowing Down Kidney Disease*, aimed at the Native American community with Native American patients telling their stories. Most of the people in the DVD were from the Salt River and the Gila River Indian Communities.

I learned from the Indian Health Services' {HIS} Dr. Charles Rhodes, the Director of their Diabetes Prevention Program, {since retired} that each tribe has been granted a percentage of a $150,000 grant for diabetes education and prevention. Not all the tribes have decided to use the money for educational purposes; some use it for treatment.

When I spoke with Dr. Andrew Narva, Director of The National Kidney Disease Education Program at the Division Of Kidney, Urologic, & Hematologic Diseases of at The National Institute of Diabetes and Digestive and Kidney Diseases which is part of the NIH and U.S. Department of Health and Human Services, he explained that I may have missed the existence of many of the CKD education programs because they were under the auspices of the Diabetes Prevention and Education programs on the reservations.

I know, I'll write about the Chronic Kidney Disease support groups I've found on Facebook. First, I will warn you that certain groups and people - not included in my list - are not real. Well, I suppose they are real people but they are posing as other people in order to make themselves more acceptable to their perceived buyers so they can sell Chinese herbal medicine.

There is quite a bit wrong with that. I find the obvious deceit insulting. Herbs themselves may be very effective, but as CKD patients we may need to take less of them since our kidneys cannot filter them out as well as non-CKD patients' kidneys can. In addition, what may be healthful for non-CKD patients is not necessarily healthful for CKD patients. Just ask your nutritionist about eating the traditional healthy diet. So many of those foods are really hard on the kidneys. It's the same principle here.

Now, the groups. Please remember you may be happy with one group, but not another. Also, some of the groups are closed and you need to seek permission to join. Contact the administrators about that. The best part of these groups is that they are all truly patients and usually run disclaimers or statements letting you know they are not doctors and you need to contact your nephrologist before you follow any of their advice.

Ready? Then keep in mind that these are in no particular order and all welcome CKD patients.

- ***Kidney Disease and Diet Ideas and Help 1***
- ***Show Your Scars Tour***
- ***Kidney Disease Is Not a Joke***
- ***The Transplant Community Outreach*** {I write *Kidney Matters* for them at their request.}
- ***Renal Patient Support Group***
- ***Chronic Kidney Disease***
- ***P2P {Peer To Peer}***
- ***But You Don't Look Sick***
- ***TCO Women's Health***
- ***Kidney Disease Shout Board***
- ***Support for Those Affected by Kidney Disease***
- ***What Is It and How Did I Get It? Early Stage Chronic Kidney Disease Experiences*** {Like how I snuck that in at the end of the list?}

Check Facebook for loads more new support groups.

Some of these groups seem to be for other kinds of patients, but I've found each of them welcoming. Some seem 'dead,' but pick up in a short time. Others that are going strong as I write may not be around by the time you get around to reading the blog. It's just reassuring to know there are other CKD patients out there to share you angst, glories, numbers, and experiences with. Try each group to find a few you like.

Did She Say Spaghetti?

7/1/13 So what will I write about? I think you already know. Dr. Wile has sent me the slide show with her wonderful visual analogies of how Chronic Kidney Disease works. We may have to back up a little.

"You already know the kidneys do important jobs for your body, like filtering your blood every 30 minutes, regulating the fluid balance in the body, providing vital hormones, producing erythropoietin (e.g. This spurs red blood cell production.), and producing the renin that regulates blood pressure."

The quote is from **What Is It and How Did I Get It? Early Stage Chronic Kidney Disease** and the e.g. from the glossary of the same.

There have been many attempts to explain how Chronic Kidney Disease impedes the kidneys' abilities to do these jobs and all the others it is tasked with. The scientific explanation leaves me scratching my head. Even as a research savvy person, there are too many terms to look up and then try to string the definitions together in some kind of coherent whole. The simplistic versions leave me frustrated that they don't say much. I've seen visuals that sort of help, but aren't quite on the mark.

Dr. Wile thought of simply using a colander draining spaghetti as a visual. Bingo! Even if you haven't cooked spaghetti yourself, you've seen it cooked. Colanders are common in the households of many different ethnic groups. The holes in the colander are akin to your kidneys' nephrons. Those are the part of the kidneys that purify and filter the blood. If a hole in the colander is closed off, or if your nephron is no longer functional, both the colander and your kidneys will not do the best job. Close off more holes or nephrons and you will have even less filtering. Hike up that number and the colander and kidneys become less and less effective. You'll end up with soggy spaghetti or Chronic Kidney Disease.

You can wash your colander for better straining. You can't do that to your kidneys. Once a nephron is dead, it's dead. Sayonara, good bye, adios. You can't bring it back to life. Before you panic, remember you have one million nephrons in each of your two kidneys. The name of the game here is: slow it down, slow down gathering those clogged holes in your colander, slow down the death rate for your nephrons.

I know it sounds like an impossible task but it isn't. You may have to make lifestyle changes such as no longer smoking and cutting down – or out – your drinking. You've got a renal diet or, at least, the name of the renal dietician the U.S. government is providing for you, call the number and make an appointment. If you have your renal diet, read it, make certain you understand it, and follow it. What about sleep? Are you making certain you're getting enough? And then there's the ever present exercise. Lately there have been studies that indicate stress can exacerbate CKD. Find new ways to deal with that, ways that work for you.

There's no one way to do any of the above, but the point is you've got to do it. Sometimes it's as annoying as... well, whatever is the most annoying thing you can think of, but it is so worth it.

You, You're Driving Me Crazy: Dedicated to Vitamin D

7/8/13   I hereby declare today Vitamin D Day. Why? Well, you see, I had this question from a reader about the conflicting reports on the value of taking supplemental vitamin D. I had hoped my research would have some kind of defining conclusion. Hah! Be prepared to have your head spin.

Last October I read a New York Times blog by Nicholas Bakalar regarding a study questioning vitamin D supplementation. According to University of Aberdeen's senior lecturer and leader of the study, Helen M. McDonald,

"The study actually shows that vitamin D does not protect you against heart disease...."

That sounds straight forward enough. However, the study also discovered no effects on C-reactive protein {a protein in the blood which may indicate artery inflammation}, LDL {low density lipoprotein - the kind that forms blockages in your arteries}, HDL {high density lipoprotein which cleans out the blockages just mentioned}, total cholesterol {all the fat in your blood}, triglycerides the major form of fat the body stores}, insulin production, or blood pressure. Whoa, ladies and gentlemen. That is quite an array of areas there.

Wait a minute. In November of last year, Washington University School of Medicine published a study in the *Journal of Biological Chemistry* that indicates vitamin D could prevent atherosclerosis {clogged arteries}, an important aspect of heart health, in diabetics. The authors of the study, Dr. Amy E. Riek and Dr. Carlos Bernal-Mizrachi, made a point of saying they did not know if vitamin D is capable of reversing atherosclerosis in diabetics. But doesn't that contradict the previous article's finding that vitamin D's effect on diabetes is questionable?

 In a more germane article printed that same month, Loyola University Health System announced that under the Institute of Medicine's new guidelines, only 35.4 % of Chronic Kidney Disease sufferers would be deemed as having insufficient levels of vitamin D rather than the 76.5% under the older guidelines. These numbers are based on a survey of patients. Keep in mind that CKD has been linked to low vitamin D levels.

The percentage of healthy people who would no longer be considered as having insufficient levels of vitamin D would also drop by more than half. Here's the kicker: while it is accepted that vitamin D is needed for your bones, there is a question about its role in …cancer, heart disease {That's what the blog above discussed.}, autoimmune diseases and diabetes {what the study above deals with}….

What concerns me is that too much vitamin D can adversely affect the heart AND the kidneys. This article was a bit more medical in terminology than I'm comfortable with.

In March of this year, the *Journal of the American Society of Nephrology* published a study stating:

"Vitamin D supplements may help maintain kidney function in transplant recipients."

Okay, so with the new guidelines you may be one of the close to 50% of Chronic Kidney Disease sufferers who no longer need vitamin D supplementation… until you receive a transplant??

While you read this particular paragraph, keep the first study in mind – the one that decided vitamin D supplemental had no effect on blood pressure.

In April, I read a NPR {National Public Radio} blog about The Brigham and Women's Hospital's small study with Blacks as their subjects. This one found that vitamin D may lessen the risks of high blood pressure in Blacks. Notice none of the other studies mentioned Blacks. I really like this one because Blacks have a higher incidence of Chronic Kidney Disease and, as we know, high blood pressure is one of the leading causes of CKD.

Concerning diabetes, another New York Times blog by the same author as the first one states,

"A new study has found a strong correlation between low vitamin D blood levels and Type 1 diabetes."

Later in the blog, one of the authors of the study made a connection between Type 1 diabetes and other diseases that are prevented by vitamin supplements. This was published the same month that the first EurekAlert.org article which stated the opposite was.

While we're on the topic of diabetes, on February 5th of this year, Nick Tate wrote on the News Max Health site,

"New Harvard University research has found that adequate levels of the 'sunshine vitamin' cut the odds of developing adult-onset type 1 diabetes by half."

I wonder if he's using the Institute of Medicine's new guidelines? And what about the same Institute of Medicine's claim that vitamin D's role in diabetes is questionable? This study was funded by the National Institute of Neurological Disorders and Stroke.

So now we leave heart disease, Chronic Kidney Disease, diabetes, and transplantation to move down to the knees. I have never heard that vitamin D can help with arthritic knees, but apparently others have. In July of this year, Medpage Today referred to an article published on January 8th. It discusses a Brigham and Women's Hospital 2-year trial contradicts observational studies that had suggested higher levels of vitamin D might slow the progression the disease {knee osteoarthritis}.

Since I am one of the lucky ones {Notice the dripping sarcasm.} to enjoy this disease, I was surprised to come across this trial. I do acknowledge the connection between vitamin D and bone health, but never thought of it as something to reverse bone damage.

Back to D

7/15/13   The following definition is from MedlinePlus. This is a service of the U.S. National Library of Medicine National Institutes of Health which I trust and often cite in the blog.

"Vitamin D helps the body absorb calcium. Calcium and phosphate are two minerals that are essential for normal bone formation. Throughout childhood, your body uses these minerals to produce bones. If you do not get enough calcium, or if your body does not absorb enough calcium from your diet, bone production and bone tissues may suffer.

Vitamin D deficiency can lead to osteoporosis in adults or rickets in children."

So, as adults, we basically need vitamin D to keep our bones healthy, although it does perform other functions such as,

"regulates calcium and phosphorous blood levels … affects the immune system."

This last definition is from the glossary of **What Is It and How Did I Get It? Early Stage Chronic Kidney Disease**.

I did manage to find out why my former nephrologist recommended supplemental vitamin D for me. Apparently, vitamin D is routinely recommended for those over 60 since – statistically speaking – more than half the people in this age group have a vitamin D deficiency. Once you are tested, the level of the vitamin D in your blood determines whether you will be advised to take a low or high dose supplement. While the normal acceptable range is 30 to 100 {depending upon which lab you use}, mine was 29 back in 2009 when I started taking the supplements. It did go up to 31 six months later. I still take the supplements to make certain it stays within range. 31 is so low in the acceptable range.

Medpage Today ran an article discussing why low vitamin D levels in whites can lead to a heart risk, but the same low vitamin D levels don't lead to heart risks in Blacks or Hispanics. I especially like Dr. Keith Norris's comment on this.

"...reinforces what we're seeing in medicine, [which] is a push toward personalized medicine where we're really looking beyond what happens to a whole group of people, but how do we understand what's happening at more [of] an individual level."

In other words, a person is a person is a person – even when it comes to their health. While there was no risk of heart disease due to low levels of vitamin D in Blacks, supplements could possibly lower blood pressure just a bit in Blacks. So, if you don't take them for one reason, you take them for another, I guess. The researchers themselves are not certain, however, whether this study was long enough to prove anything.

Before you get down in the mouth about this information, let's talk about vitamin D in kidney patients and gum disease {Get it? down in the mouth? gum disease? oh well.} This time, the information is specifically for those with Chronic Kidney Disease. According to Dr. Jessica Bastos back in April of this year:

"This association seems to be mediated through an impairment in clearing bacterial infection due to a decrease in cathelicidin {Antimicrobial polypeptides} production."

There is a purported correlation between low levels of vitamin D and low levels of cathelicidin production. I don't know about you, but I intend to print the blog and check that I took my vitamin D today. My dentist is a nice guy, but this is my mouth we're talking about.

I have many more articles in front of me, so I'm going to simply list the areas in which low vitamin D is involved.
- cardiovascular
- Chronic Kidney Disease {the purpose of this blog, lest we forget}
- health hip fracture risk
- hepatitis B {Have you decided to take the inoculation against this?}
- hypertension
- stroke

Got how dangerous low levels of vitamin D can be? Good. Be ready to be confounded. Another study links low levels of vitamin D with long life. The studies suggest that low serum levels of vitamin D are a consequence, rather than a cause of, disease according to its authors.

Oh, the Gall!

7/22/13   My daughter's cholecystectomy is taking precedence in my mind. Her what, you ask? That, my friends, is what the procedure to remove your gallbladder is called. By the way, I asked what it was, too.

This is Nima's description of how it all started and what the procedure was like.

"At one point or another we've all that had that midnight snack of a slice of cold pizza and maybe some juice to wash it down. So when I woke up with severe sharp pain on my right side I didn't think much of it, except I shouldn't have eaten that pizza, and where is the Tums?

After two Tums and a hot shower, the sharp pain continued all around the middle of my back to the middle of my front right side. I finally thought to myself, 'Don't be stupid. You have a family history of CKD, and one family member who passed stones a few years back. Better to be safe than sorry, get it checked.'

Off to the ER I went. After I described my symptoms to the first year resident, she picked up very quickly on the fact it could be gallstone/gallbladder related due to the side of the pain (right) and asked for a urine sample, as well as ordering blood work, and a sonogram of that area. I was also given an IV, morphine drip for pain (which honestly did nothing – too much pain- all I wanted to do was rock back and forth or keep walking in circles to help me be in motion so I didn't have to think about the pain), and eventually antibiotics.

The doctor came back with the results of the blood work to tell me that my white blood count was elevated to 12, an indication the gallbladder was infected. I was finally taken to sonogram. A bariatric first year resident explained I had an impassable 2.7 in. diameter gallstone that was causing blockage in the duct in the front and a bunch of pain. There'd be no way to take it out other than surgery. After meeting with the attending physician, he concurred. He also mentioned that, because the gallbladder was infected, it'd be smart to remove it.

So, I did. I'll now have to learn an entirely new way to eat (low-fat) as the gallbladder is what processes fat. I've learned quickly if I consume the slightest bit of fat, my body's response is 'Um, what the hell are we supposed to do with that?!' and to reject it in a not so nice way. I'll have to play it smart and step up the exercise and water intake as well to make up for the missing organ and amount of bile that could now possibly be floating in my body because it has nowhere to go. As for pizza at midnight? Well unless, I want another episode like the one I just had, those days are now in my rearview mirror."

After speaking with my daughter, I still wondered what gallstones have to do with Chronic Kidney Disease? Searching the web only garnered this one article from January, 2009 – that's four and a half years ago – and the study only covered Taiwan. Of course, I found it at the National Institutes of Health.

"The prevalence of gallbladder stones in patients with Chronic Kidney Disease is significantly higher than in those without Chronic Kidney Disease. Our findings suggest that increasing age, Chronic Kidney Disease, body mass index > or =27 kg/m {greater than 59 pounds}, metabolic syndrome, and cirrhosis are the related factors for gallbladder stone formation."

Now think about it another way: you already have a compromised immune system because you have CKD. Gallstones can cause infection of the gallbladder. As in Nima's experience, infection causes white blood cell elevation. So you know you have an infection, you might even realize it could be in the bile ducts, too. But did you check to see if there's infection in other areas of your body? That would mean you can read your own test results or have the kind of relationship with your doctors – especially your nephrologist – to freely ask questions.

As for what this organ does, this is what Medline had to say.

"The gallbladder is a pear-shaped organ under your liver. It stores bile, a fluid made by your liver to digest fat. As your stomach and intestines digest food, your gallbladder releases bile through a tube called the common bile duct. The duct connects your gallbladder and liver to your small intestine."

Keep in mind that your liver, the largest organ in your body {The skin is actually the largest organ, but it's external.} is the other organ that filters your blood. Since your CKD has been diagnosed, your liver is already working harder. Add losing your gallbladder and you've got one very hard working – possibly overworked? – liver.

What about the surgery, you ask? There are two kinds: open which is surgery as we understood it before laparoscopic surgery and laparoscopic surgery. In the latter kind,

"Under general anesthesia, so the patient is asleep throughout the procedure.

- Using a cannula (a narrow tube-like instrument), the surgeon enters the abdomen in the area of the belly-button.
- A laparoscope (a tiny telescope) connected to a special camera is inserted through the cannula, giving the surgeon a magnified view of the patient's internal organs on a television screen.
- Other cannulas are inserted which allow your surgeon to delicately separate the gallbladder from its attachments and then remove it through one of the openings.
- Many surgeons perform an X-ray, called a cholangiogram, to identify stones, which may be located in the bile channels, or to insure that structures have been identified.
- If the surgeon finds one or more stones in the common bile duct, (s)he may remove them with a special scope, may choose to have them removed later through a second minimally invasive procedure, or may convert to an open operation in order to remove all the stones during the operation.

After the surgeon removes the gallbladder, the small incisions are closed with a stitch or two or with surgical tape."

Thank you for this information *Society of American Gastrointestinal and Endoscopic Surgeons.*

*Nima did ask me to tell you that she experienced quite a bit of gas after the surgery and suggested that you, as a CKD patient, arm yourself before you go into surgery with the knowledge of what you can take for gas.

The Eyes Have It

7/29/13   I have gotten lots of questions about what macular degeneration is. It's an eye problem. The macula {Macular means about the macula.} is the layer of tissue on the back of the inside of your eyeball in the middle of your retina. The National Institute of Health's Senior Health has a succinct definition of the disease.

"Age-related macular degeneration, also known as AMD, is an eye disease that affects the macula, a part of the retina. The retina sends light from the eye to the brain, and the macula allows you to see fine detail."

No one seems to know why it happens, but it does get worse as you get older. There are two kinds. Lucky me, I have the dry or non-neovascular or nonexudative kind. Nonvascular means NOT new blood vessels, which is the wet or vascular kind of macular degeneration.

As for exudative, the medical dictionary at The Free Dictionary, explains that exudation means,

"the escape of fluid, cells, and cellular debris from blood vessels and their deposition in or on the tissues, usually as the result of inflammation."

Again, I have the nonexudative kind. So wet macular degeneration – the kind I do not have – consists of fluid escaping from the eyeball to form new blood vessels. I'm going to let Natural Products That Make a Difference handle this one since their explanation is both clear and succinct.

"Wet Macular Degeneration (also called neovascular or exudative) refers to a condition where the macula degenerates (just as in Dry Macular Degeneration), but as a result of hemorrhaging blood vessels in the eye or the abnormal growth of blood vessels in the eye. In Wet Macular Degeneration, abnormal blood vessel growth is triggered in the choriocapillaries (behind the retina) resulting in the leakage of blood and protein. The resulting fluid leakage and overgrowth of blood vessels can quickly damage the macula and its rod and cone cells, resulting in severe loss of central vision. Hemorrhaging of the blood vessels around the retina or macula can cause vision loss virtually overnight, much the same way Diabetic Retinopathy does. Even if the vessels do not hemorrhage, the growth of blood vessels on the macula or the retina can cause severe central vision loss (though this may not be as sudden)."

This may be corrected by surgery, something that is not available to dry macular degeneration sufferers. That's where the sarcastic "Lucky me" came in above. However, you could also lose your vision overnight with this kind, so maybe I am lucky that I have the dry kind.

Dry macular degeneration is caused by drusen or yellow deposits made up of lipids {ph no, a fatty protein!} Of course, there has to be two kinds of these as well, hard and soft. The hard doesn't seem to be problematic, or at least not for a long time, but the soft? This one is a good indication you have AMD or Age-Related Macular Degeneration.

The soft drusen tend to cluster together and, with no distinct borders, it makes sense that would affect your vision. Diagnosing does require your ophthalmologist perform a dilated eye examination. Now remember, no one knows what causes AMD so drusen are not the source, simply an indication of higher risk.

No surgery fix for me since I have dry macular degeneration, but according to the second Age Related Eye Disease Study or AREDS2 study, certain vitamins and minerals might slow down the rate of degeneration by 25%. I don't know about you, but I'll take even a 25% chance. These are my eyes!

My ophthalmologist had a formula made just for this purpose and wanted me to take it. Of course he did. He's my ophthalmologist and my eyes are his first priority. But, while I value them greatly, I made it clear my kidneys are my first priority. This is where the Chronic Kidney Disease element comes into today's blog.

I'd had kidney stones, so I couldn't take the vitamin C in the formula. There's no kidney related reason not to take vitamin A, but it is included for the purpose of avoiding cataracts. I've already had cataract surgery so it wouldn't do me any good. Same for vitamin E.

Zinc was in the formula, but this metal – which is an essential trace element – contains cadmium which may cause kidney failure. Goodbye zinc. Copper, another metal and essential trace element, was in the formula because zinc supplements can be the cause of copper deficiency. One problem. Copper can cause kidney damage if you take large quantities or take it over a long period of time. Can't take that.

And then there was Omega 3 Fish Oil, but I already take that to reduce the progress of my Chronic Kidney Disease and in larger quantities than suggested by the ARED2 study. The antioxidants {inhibits the negative effects of oxidation} lutein and zeaxanthin are also in the formula and I am taking them separately. I looked them up on WebMD before I made my decision. This is what I found there.

"Eye-related benefits: Lutein and zeaxanthin protect the eyes from harmful high-energy light waves, such as some ultraviolet rays in sunlight. Studies suggest that high levels of lutein and zeaxanthin in eye tissue are associated with better vision, especially in dim light or where glare is a problem."

There were many more ingredients in this ophthalmologist's formula and I'm beginning to understand that each ophthalmologist may slightly alter the formula he has made for his dry macular degeneration patients. This degeneration process could take up to 10 years... or less, much less.

It's Not Just for Eating

8/12/13   I'm eager to get into today's topic: liver, or rather fatty liver disease. I vaguely remember this showing up on an MRI some time ago and my primary care physician telling me about it. That's when I was obsessed with weight since my nephrologist had just explained I would do better at slowing down the progress of the CKD if I lost weight. My first response to my PCP? "That's fat, too?"

Once she stopped laughing, she explained that many people have fatty livers but you have to be careful about it before you end up with {in my case} NAFLD or Non-Alcoholic Fatty Liver Disease.

So, we know fat gets deposited in the liver and too much is no good. The question is how much is too much? According to WebMD
Some fat in the liver is normal. But if fat makes up more than 5%-10% of the weight of your liver, you may have alcoholic or nonalcoholic liver disease. In some cases, these diseases can lead to serious complications.

Let's backtrack a little to find out why the liver is important in the first place. According to The Mayo Clinic, these are the functions of the liver.

- Breaking down harmful substances
- Removing waste products from the blood
- Storing nutrients and vitamins
- Moderating chemical levels in the body

Take a look at the second function again. Does it sound familiar? Yep, that's one of the functions of your kidneys, your not functioning at capacity kidneys. You're already having trouble because one of your organs can't do its job adequately, you certainly don't need an additional organ responsible for the same job to be compromised. Ah, that must be why I'm writing about fatty liver disease on a Chronic Kidney Disease blog.

By the way, a liver specialist is called a hepatologist.   That comes from the same word root as hepatitis. Remember I'd urged you to make certain you took the series of hepatitis B inoculations since your kidneys are already comprised? And suggested you might want to be checked for any hepatitis C in your blood work? Hepatitis is from the same Greek word root, hepa, which means liver.

Okay, maybe we need to know a little more about the liver. It's a large organ, in fact, the second largest in your body. You'll find yours under your rib cage on the right side of your body. It's shaped sort of like a football that's flat on one side. Oh, yes, weight: three pounds.

Like CKD, NAFLD or Non-Alcoholic Fatty Liver Disease is mostly a silent disease; it usually has no symptoms. When symptoms do occur, it seems to me that they would be hard to pin down as NAFLD since not an array of these symptoms is needed for a diagnose, but any one of them will suffice... but then again, I'm not a doctor.

"fatigue, weakness, weight loss, loss of appetite, nausea, abdominal pain, spider-like blood vessels, jaundice, itching, edema, ascites {Swelling of the abdomen} and mental confusion."

Thank you to the American Liver Foundation. This is from their nifty little fact sheet that is simple to understand.

Then I got to wondering about why this disease could be dangerous. It's the possible progression that makes it dangerous. You're told you have a fatty liver {AFLD is fatty liver disease caused by alcoholism}, you don't lose weight {If you're overweight or obese}, lower your cholesterol and triglycerides, control your diabetes {If you have it} or avoid alcohol, and the disease worsens.

Your liver swells. This is called steatohepatitis. That may cause cirrhosis or scarring over a long period. The cirrhosis could eventually cause liver cancer or failure. The saddest part of all this is that some people develop NAFLD or AFLD for no reason at all.

The good part {There's a good part?} is that a healthy diet and regular exercise – just like CKD, isn't it? – may prevent scarring or even reverse it if the disease is caught early enough. Since there usually aren't any symptoms, fatty liver disease is most often uncovered by your usual blood tests. A high level of liver enzymes could be the tip off.

Spurs in Arizona

8/19/13 Of course there are spurs in Arizona, you may find yourself thinking... and you're right. Both kinds are in abundance here. Both kinds? Sure, the ones you wear on your boots and the ones you wear in your boots, actually inside your foot.

I recently had pain in my heel and figured it was just another sign that I'm growing older {Funny, I do that every year}. When I casually mentioned this to my ever vigilant primary care doctor, she pounced. She's so good at that and since she's the one who uncovered my Chronic Kidney Disease, I listen when she pounces.

An order for three different foot x-rays revealed a formerly broken little toe {judo, pre-pregnancy, 33 years ago}, osteoarthritis {That's like telling a painfully sun burned person they're sun burned} and a heel bone spur. A what? Oh, an osteophyte! Osteo comes from the Latin *osseus—os, ossis* meaning bone and the Greek *osteon*, also meaning bone. {Thank you for the memory, Hunter College of the City University of New York course in Greek and Latin roots taken a zillion years ago.}

You know the name of my book about Chronic Kidney Disease is ***What Is It and How Did I Get It? Early Stage Chronic Kidney Disease***. That's become my approach to any new ailment that shows up for me. And there are lots of those lately.

We know from its name that a bone spur has to do with the bone. We also know what a spur is. Try to visualize a spur on the end of your heel. According to MedicineNet:

"Heel spur: A bony spur projecting from the back or underside of the heel that often makes walking painful. Spurs at the back of the heel are associated with inflammation of the Achilles tendon (Achilles tendinitis) and cause tenderness and pain at the back of the heel that is made worse by pushing off the ball of the foot. Spurs under the sole (plantar area) are associated with inflammation of the plantar fascia (the 'bowstring-like' tissue stretching from the heel underneath the sole) and cause localized tenderness and pain made worse by stepping down on the heel."

The latter is my problem. I'd actually thought that dancing was magic because when I did at Sustainable Blues Phoenix, I didn't feel any pain at all. Turns out that's because I was dancing on my toes, not my heels. I've still got to thank daughter, Abby Wegerski, and her co-instructor for those two pain free hours a week.

On to how I got it. WebMD tells us,

"Heel spurs occur when calcium deposits build up on the underside of the heel bone, a process that usually occurs over a period of many months. Heel spurs are often caused by strains on foot muscles and ligaments, stretching of the plantar fascia, and repeated tearing of the membrane that covers the heel bone. Heel spurs are especially common among athletes whose activities include large amounts of running and jumping."

I don't run and I don't jump, but I do pop in a walking tape DVD every other day or so. Could that be the cause? I read on only to discover that age, weight, walking gait, worn out shoes {I wear the comfortable ones until they literally fall apart.} and "frequent short bursts of physical activity" could be the culprits. I am pretty sedentary except for those exercise periods each day.

Still not satisfied, I wanted to know what I could do about the heel spur I'd developed. Dr. Andrew Weil, my health hero before I developed Chronic Kidney Disease has quite a lot to say about that.

"….Symptomatic treatment involves rest, especially from the activity that is contributing to the condition and making symptoms worse …. Ice is recommended immediately following it…. Stretching exercises that gently lengthen the calm muscle will relax the tissue surrounding the heel and should be done several times a day, especially in the morning and after prolonged sitting. Over-the-counter or prescription-strength anti-inflammatory medications can help temporarily…. Deep tissue massage, taping and other physical therapy modalities can also be helpful. Arch support is highly recommended, either with shoe inserts or custom orthotics made by podiatrists. If pain continues, a steroid injection at the site of pain may be recommended….Sometimes bone spurs can be surgically removed or an operation to loosen the fascia – called a plantar fascia release – can be performed."

I urge you to read his article for yourself since I omitted many of his warnings due to lack of space. They are valid. He also suggests natural remedies that you may find helpful, but be careful about the herbs. As CKD patients, we need to rely on tested substances and, often, herbal supplements are not. It was so much easier to deal with my health before CKD, or so I thought. As CKD patients, we cannot take Over the Counter (OTC) pain relievers.

Heel that Pain made a common sense point, although they sell the product to follow the common sense. I am not endorsing their product because I haven't tried it, but I do use orthotics from several different companies.

"The heel spur, because it is part of the bone, actually has no feeling in it. The pain that is generated from the heel spur is due to the soft tissue around the heel spur that gets irritated and inflamed and bruised. This is what creates the heel pain from the spur itself. If you can properly support the heel bone so that friction and motion are reduced, it will allow the soft tissue around the area of the heel spur to heal, and have a reduction in the inflammation and tenderness. The goal would be to support the heel bone enough so that the heel spur does not dig into the soft tissue."

Wait a minute… I think I remember that I have spinal bone spurs too. Well, there's next week's blog.

She Can Really DISH It Out!

8/26/13   I write about all these ailments I have, but I need to re-focus you here. They're all small or just beginning for me so I'm not in any dire straits. Even the Chronic Kidney Disease is holding steady at Stage 3. I didn't want you to think I was falling apart at the seams…which is kind of an opposite analogy for how I am very slowly falling apart internally, anyway.

I promised to write about D.I.S.H. {Diffuse Idiopathic Skeletal Hyperostosis} today, so I'll start at the beginning. Soon after our wedding, we took an overnight trip to Biosphere 2 in Tucson, Arizona. It was every bit as interesting as I'd hoped it would be, but I came home really ill. The diagnoses were flying all over the medical map, but a CAT scan at John C. Lincoln Health Network discovered something entirely unrelated that I hadn't known about.

BONY THORAX: Large hypertrophic spurs throughout the lower dorsal spine suggest the possibility of DISH.

What? The what? Oh, the thorax. That's:

"The part of the human body between the neck and the diaphragm, partially encased by the ribs and containing the heart and lungs; the chest"

according to The Free Dictionary. That made sense since that's what hurt, but I couldn't help thinking of a fish's dorsal fin when I read "lower dorsal spine."

So, as usual, I looked it up. Biology online told me it is,

"One of the three distinct portions along the spine or the vertebral column (the other two are the cervical spine and the lumbar spine), and is the longest section comprised of twelve thoracic vertebrae that house the spinal cord along the rachidian channel."

Great. I was lost. What did I know about rachidian channels? And where on the spine was it?

I found discussions of rachidian channels on the internet, but I couldn't follow them. Maybe it would help to further break down the definition. In a reference dictionary, I found that, among other definitions, dorsal means

"situated on or toward the upper side of the body, equivalent to the back, or posterior, in humans."

Wait a minute, so there was something on the lower back of my spine. Got it.

I know from last week's blog {and so do you} what bone spurs are, so now I just need to define hypertrophic.   Back to my college Greek and Latin roots: hyper means over, above, excessive. Trophic sounded familiar, but I just wasn't sure. I decided it would make more sense to research the word as a whole and discovered this definition at Dictionary Reference

"abnormal enlargement of a part or organ; excessive growth."

I should have figured. There were bone spurs on the back of my lower spine. Ugh! Another indication of my advanced {Can I get away with writing advancing instead?} age.

But, there's more folks! Don't touch that dial! This suggested D.I.S.H. I went right to my old friend The Mayo Clinic for clarification.

"Diffuse idiopathic skeletal hyperostosis (DISH) is calcification or a bony hardening of ligaments in areas where they attach to your spine. Also known as Forestier's disease, diffuse idiopathic skeletal hyperostosis may cause no symptoms and require no treatment. The most common symptoms are mild to moderate pain and stiffness in your upper back. DISH may also affect your neck and lower back. Some people experience DISH in other areas, such as shoulders, elbows, knees and heels.

DISH can be progressive. As it worsens, DISH can cause serious complications."

Being thorough, I looked up Forestier's disease, too. This is what MedTerms had to say about it.

"A form of degenerative arthritis characteristically associated with flowing calcification along the sides of the vertebrae of the spine and commonly with inflammation (tendinitis) and calcification of the tendons at their attachments points to bone.

Because areas of the spine and tendons can become inflamed, nonsteroidal anti-inflammatory drugs (NSAIDs) such as ibuprofen can be helpful in relieving both pain and inflammation."

Makes sense. I have arthritis {in my case, degenerative inflammation of the joints} everywhere else in my body, why not my spine too? But the jokes on me. Notice that NSAIDS can be helpful. Yep, Chronic Kidney Disease sufferers cannot take NSAIDS. I'm lucky that I had a high pain tolerance before the CKD and, it seems to me, that it's been rising ever since my diagnose five years ago. If you can't take anything for the pain, you learn to live with as much pain as you can.

I'm uncomfortable sometimes, I can no longer exercise the way I want to for as long as and hard as I want to, but I can dance! I'm thankful because that's what makes me happy anyway. Now, if I could only find a way to dance 24/7....

A1C! A1C! (Sounds like a Cheer to Me!)

9/2/13 Let's start the way we usually do with a definition. I picked up Amgen's ***Understanding Your Lab Values: A guide for patients with Chronic Kidney Disease***. While this is a drug company {And I don't recommend any drugs; that's up to your doctor}, their informational guides are usually clear and straight to the point. They define A1C as:

"a test that measures your average blood glucose levels over 2 to 3 months."

Mine is evaluated as per my usual quarterly blood draw.

You've probably figured out that this has to do with diabetes or pre-diabetes. According to DaVita, people with Chronic Kidney Disease should keep their A1C readings between 4.0 and 5.9%. Mine has been rising steadily for the last several years and is presently at 6.1, which is considered pre-diabetic.

Okay, so your glucose levels can be tested for a two to three month average and over a certain percentage is considered pre-diabetic. What is so important about blood glucose anyway?

Our old friend MedicineNet tells us blood glucose is,

"The main sugar that the body makes from the food in the diet. Glucose is carried through the bloodstream to provide energy to all cells in the body. Cells cannot use glucose without the help of insulin. Glucose is a simple sugar (a monosaccharide). The body produces it from protein, fat and, in largest part, carbohydrate. Ingested glucose is absorbed directly into the blood from the intestine and results in a rapid increase in blood glucose. Glucose is also known as dextrose."

Got it! We need blood glucose for energy. And the cells need insulin to provide this energy from glucose. Well, how is this a problem? Wait a minute – insulin – diabetes. Oh, my!

I'm getting close to diabetes. All right, then let's look at diabetes. What's that? Well, we can figure out it's the body's inability to handle a surplus of glucose in the body, but what harm is it specifically to you {and me} as a Chronic Kidney Disease patient?

According to Diabetes.co.uk,

"The kidneys are another organ that is at particular risk of damage as a result of diabetes and the risk is again increased by poorly controlled diabetes, high blood pressure and cholesterol."

I am not liking this. I'm already being treated for hypertension {high blood pressure} and hyperlipidemia {high cholesterol}. I don't think I can afford to add diabetes to the list. And that's why next week's blog will be about diabetes.

You Mean It's Really The Carbs?

9/9/13 When I think of diabetes, or pre-diabetes, I think of sugar. Your A1C measures the percentage of blood glucose {Think sugar.} in you, so I just presumed that's why it was used to determine if you have diabetes. Last week, when I was researching this test, I came across material suggesting it was carbohydrates – not the sugar I had assumed – that needs to be cut down in an effort to slow down the disease.

As usual, I'm getting a little ahead of myself. I think I've discovered a formula that works when explaining… and it starts with a definition. According to Medical News Today:

"Diabetes, often referred to by doctors as diabetes mellitus, describes a group of metabolic diseases in which the person has high blood glucose (blood sugar), either because insulin production is inadequate, or because the body's cells do not respond properly to insulin, or both. Patients with high blood sugar will typically experience polyuria (frequent urination), they will become increasingly thirsty (polydipsia) and hungry (polyphagia)."

Mellitus comes from the Latin and refers to sugar sweetened. Notice that diabetes is often called Diabetes Mellitus. Hmmm, another reason I thought it was ingested sugar that causes the disease. Yet, it is described as a metabolic disease; that is, a disease that deals with our metabolism – the way we process the foods we eat to gain energy.

Well then, where does insulin come in? Just in case you forgot, MedicineNet tells us insulin is:

"A natural hormone made by the pancreas that controls the level of the sugar glucose in the blood. Insulin permits cells to use glucose for energy. Cells cannot utilize glucose without insulin."

Oh, so if your body is not producing enough insulin   or none at all - or the cells can't respond to the insulin produced in the usual way, the energy from the blood glucose can't be used to provide energy for your cells. Accepted. But isn't blood sugar still sugar, say from candy, cake, cookies and the like? You know, the things we don't eat as Chronic Kidney Disease patients.

Well… yes and no. Certainly these food items contain sugar. That's part of what makes them so delicious. But they are also carbohydrates, a word I usually associate with bread and pasta. MedicineNet's definition of carbohydrate cleared up my confusion.

"One of the three nutrient compounds, along with fat and protein, used as energy sources (calories) by the body. Carbohydrates take the form of simple sugars or of more complex forms, such as starches and fiber. Complex carbohydrates come naturally from plants. Intake of complex carbohydrates, when they are substituted for saturated fat, can lower blood cholesterol. Carbohydrates produce 4 calories of energy per gram. When eaten, all carbohydrates are broken down into the sugar glucose."

Ahh! So all carbohydrates, whether from starches or sugars break down into sugar glucose. This is starting to sound familiar. When I brought my pre-diabetes to the nutritionist at my nephrologist's office, she gave me quite a bit of information and a handout from DCE, a dietetic practice group of the American Dietetic Association. Did you know that starchy vegetables, fruits, juices and milk also contain carbohydrates? It hadn't occurred to me.

Remember the way to measure a half cup or a whole cup when you don't have measuring cups but want to stay on the renal diet, including portion control? It's the size of your palm for half a cup and the size of a clenched fist for a whole cup. The same method is used to measure a portion of carbohydrates. Good for us, one less thing to learn. You know measuring cups are better, but to be honest, I got a little tired of dragging them around with me in only a few weeks.

You can also buy portion control plates on the internet, but frankly, it's just as easy to measure it {whatever it is} out once and then know what that size portion is. For example, we needed glasses so when I first used a new one, I measured the water it held and now know the new glasses hold 15 oz. unlike the blue ones we already have which hold 8 oz.

The Mayo Clinic has a good diet plan for diabetes, but it won't work for Chronic Kidney Disease patients as it is. For example, whole wheat flour raises your blood glucose less than white flour, but has too much phosphorous for us, so we are warned to avoid it. Yoghurt, cheese, beans, and nuts are no-nos on my renal diet, but are often recommended in diabetes diets.

You need to know what you can and cannot eat on your renal diet before you look at the diabetes diet so you know what to cross out immediately. This is what makes it easier for me to plan what I'll be eating that day.

You also need to space out your carbohydrates. This grand-daughter of a Jewish miller from the Ukraine really did miss sitting down to eat a whole loaf of fresh black bread at one sitting… with butter, no less. The diabetic diet isn't that bad, though: for me it's 2 to 3 carbohydrate portions at breakfast, lunch and dinner with a one carbohydrate portion at three snacks – one after each meal. As I understand it, each carbohydrate portion is 15 grams.

Statins: No Easy Decision Here

9/16/13   A reader asked me to write about this topic. Like me, she is a woman in her middle sixties who takes statins. Unlike me, she has had adverse side effects. Who even remembered about these?

Of course, I read the information handout the pharmacy attaches to the bag containing your prescription. Of course, I researched this drug on the internet when it was first prescribed for me. But that was years ago and, while I periodically re-read the pharmacy's handout, the dangers of this drug never quite resonated with me. Dangers? With statins? That's most people's reaction.

Let's go back to the beginning with an explanation of what statins are and what they do. According to MedicineNet,

"'Statins' is a class of drugs that lowers the level of cholesterol in the blood by reducing the production of cholesterol by the liver. (The other source of cholesterol in the blood is dietary cholesterol.) Statins block the enzyme in the liver that is responsible for making cholesterol."

Makes sense. But what's cholesterol? Medical News Today tells us:

"Cholesterol is a lipid (fat) which is produced by the liver. Cholesterol is vital for normal body function. Every cell in our body has cholesterol in its outer layer."

Okay, so we need this particular lipid but sometimes – between the foods we eat and our body's functioning – we produce too much of it. Then it may stick to our arteries as plaque, possibly narrowing or even blocking them. This could lead to CAD or coronary artery disease {heart problems}.

Here's the important part for Chronic Kidney Disease sufferers: it's the liver – the organ that produces cholesterol – that is affected by the statins. That's the only other filtering system your body has and your kidneys are already compromised. TWO compromised filtering systems seems like a really poor idea to me. Yet, sometimes, we need to take statins.

I went to my favorite, The Mayo Clinic, for information about when you need to be on a statin.

"If you have high cholesterol, meaning your total cholesterol level is 240 milligrams per deciliter (mg/dL) (6.22 millimoles per liter, or mmol/L) or higher, or your low-density lipoprotein cholesterol (LDL, or 'bad' cholesterol) level is 130 mg/dL (3.37 mmol/L) or higher, your doctor may recommend you begin to take a statin. But the numbers alone won't tell you or your doctor the whole story.

If the only risk factor you have is high cholesterol, you may not need medication because your risk of heart attack and stroke could otherwise be low. High cholesterol is only one of a number of risk factors for heart attack and stroke."

As CKD patients, we already have another risk factor. If, like me, those numbers mystify you, you can find them on your quarterly blood test reports which will usually have an 'H' to indicate high or 'L' to indicate low {You won't find that if you're on statins.} next to the numbers for your total cholesterol and your low-density lipoprotein levels.

As for how hyperlipidemia {high cholesterol} can affect your body and why statins are prescribed, I took a look at a non-technical explanation on Heart Disease.com.

"Clinical studies have shown that statins significantly reduce the risk of heart attack and death in patients with proven coronary artery disease (CAD), and can also reduce cardiac events in patients with high cholesterol levels who are at increased risk for heart disease. While best known as drugs that lower cholesterol, statins have several other beneficial effects that may also improve cardiac risk, and that may turn out to be even more important than their cholesterol-reducing properties."

Well, that all sounds good so what's the problem? It's the side effects, ladies and gentlemen. It's all the *may cause* that you find on the websites and in your pharmacy handout information.

I went to a new site for me, Statinseffects.org, and was staggered by the side effects.

"The risk of liver & kidney damage, muscle damage, increased risk of cancer & other side effects of cholesterol lowering drugs are good reason why exercise & diet should be patient's first resort for controlling cholesterol levels. For people who must take cholesterol lowering medications, the dose needs to be reduced to minimum by again exercise & diet. The main concern seems to be the overuse or underuse of the medication, despite of the evidence that high cholesterol level itself is not the most important factor of heart disease. It is, however, the ratio between total & HDL cholesterol levels."

You *know* what popped out at me: kidney damage. We already have kidney damage. Each of these side effects deserves a blog of its own. But, it is important to remember that these are possible, not definite, side effects.

Am I endorsing statin use for hyperlipidemia? No, I'm not. I'm not a doctor. You need to discuss this with your doctor. Mine, at the time of my diagnose with hyperlipidemia, was amenable to my desire not to take the drugs for a while.

My former PCP agreed to this in an attempt to demonstrate to me that I needed the medication. This was about six years before I was diagnosed with CKD. For three months – the acknowledged honeymoon period – my numbers were great. And then they started to climb... and climb, despite the dietary changes and exercise. I am just one of those unlucky ones with naturally high cholesterol. Try this for yourself if your doctor agrees, but keep your health foremost in your mind.

Neurology –> Neuropathy –> New To Me

9/23/13   Here's my new medical mess: neuropathy. I can't tell you how long it took for me to simply pronounce the word correctly. I knew neuro comes from the Latin for nerve and discovered that pathy, also from Latin, is a:

"word-forming element meaning feeling, suffering, emotion, disorder, disease"

{Thanks for the help on pathy goes to The Online Etymology Dictionary.} There was no connect in my brain until my family doctor sent me to a neurologist.

Why you ask? I wondered aloud in her office why I was feeling such tingling in both of my hands and, sometimes, my feet. I found no discernible pattern to the tingling, although I could tell it was stronger in the hands than the feet.

Next thing I knew, I had an appointment with a neurologist. This turned out to be a good move. It was deemed necessary to have EMGs on both my upper and lower extremities.

EMG means Electromyography. Big help, huh? Back to basics. According to eMedicineHealth,

"… electromyography involves testing the electrical activity of muscles."

Next question: why in heaven's name would anyone want to do that? I suspected it might have to do with a trapped nerve since I'd had carpal tunnel surgery 27 years ago and remembered a little bit of the process for diagnosing it.

MedicineNet.com answered that one for me.

"When muscles are active, they produce an electrical current. This current is usually proportional to the level of the muscle activity."

So did that mean I had carpal tunnel again? Oh, sorry, carpal tunnel is when the median {middle} nerve in your wrist is trapped by the ligament. Ligament surgery was pretty painful. I'm hoping things have improved in the last 27 years… just in case, you understand.

Back to why. I found an answer I could live with on my old friend The Mayo Clinic's website.

"EMG results are often necessary to help diagnose or rule out a number of conditions such as:

- Muscle disorders, such as muscular dystrophy or polymyositis
- Diseases affecting the connection between the nerve and the muscle, such as myasthenia gravis
- Disorders of nerves outside the spinal cord (peripheral nerves), such as carpal tunnel syndrome or peripheral neuropathies
- Disorders that affect the motor neurons in the brain or spinal cord, such as amyotrophic lateral sclerosis or polio
- Disorders that affect the nerve root, such as a herniated disk in the spine"

I was floored. I hadn't remembered that both my family physician and my new neurologist had explained this. I only concentrated on the possible carpal tunnel. Come to think of it, it would have had to be something else in my feet. Lesson learned: you need to keep reminding yourself to listen to your doctors' explanations even if you think you know the information already.

Rumor had it that this was a very painful test, but the neurologist distracted me with a constant stream of chatter about CKD, neurology, and families while he worked on my lower extremities. By the next day, we're weren't chattering anymore but having serious discussions. This distracted me so much that I was barely aware of what he was doing to my hands. Pain wasn't a problem during either day's testing.

Time to tell you what the good doctor actually did to me. I was asked not to use any lotions or creams the days of the tests. When we were ready to start, I was asked to lay down for the lower extremities test and sit up on the examination table for the upper extremities test.

From my side, the tests were simple. First, electrodes were applied to different parts of my legs or arms {depending on which were being tested that day}. Once he had recorded the readings from the electrodes, he pierced my skin with needles. I cannot say any of this hurt, but there was some discomfort.

Bear had the test years ago and had expected me to come home in extreme pain. Instead, I went to meet a friend for coffee one day and to an educational meeting the other. It really didn't hurt.

My neurologist gave me the results of both days' tests as well as those of the blood test he'd ordered for TSH {blood test for thyroid-stimulating hormone}, B12, folate, and vitamin D. Apparently, a deficit of any of these could cause the tingling I had. None of my readings for these elements were out of range.

What I really got a kick out of was watching him use Dragon Medical to write his notes. That's the doctors' version of the same program I've been struggling with since Christmas!

So far, I don't need anything. He suggested a follow up visit. I suggested ten years. He didn't laugh. I suggested a year. He still didn't laugh and told me six months would do. I guess being on the borderline of having carpal tunnel is more serious than I thought.

How does this impact CKD? There is medication that can help, but I didn't want to discuss it yet since it is eliminated via the kidneys. I've become pretty good at doing without medication these days. More on that should it come to a point when it's a necessity.

Deodorant Doubts

9/30/13 I've been playing around with the idea of a newsletter concerning which beauty and hygiene products are safe for Chronic Kidney Disease patients. {Feel free to 'steal' the idea.} Here's why: every day I use deodorant and every time I pick up the container I'm reminded of the warning on it:

"Ask a doctor before use if you have kidney disease."

I did just that about three years ago. At first, my nephrologist was seemingly annoyed at the question, almost as if no one had ever asked him that before. {Is that possible?} I imagine he had his P.A. check a deodorant container because he did have her call me back to say that was only for late stage CKD. Notice there's no explanation in that message and, yep, this is the nephrologist I no longer see.

Last week, I did the marketing as I usually do. Deodorant was on the list I'd written. I picked up one brand, then another, and a third. I decided to look at all the brands available and they all had that same warning. Why had I never researched this before?

Good question. I'm a firm believer in "It's never too late." Rather than a discussion of which brands are safe for those of us with kidney disease, I'll be going into the mechanics {if that's the right word} of deodorant and kidney disease.

According to Dr. Nathalie Beauchamp in a January, 2010, Ezine article, the culprit is,

"Propylene Glycol – found in thousands of cosmetic products – to help moisturize. It is also an ingredient used in anti-freeze and brake fluid, so it's no surprise that it could cause liver abnormalities and kidney damage."

But I was surprised since I'd always assumed it was the aluminum in the deodorant that was the problem. It made sense to me that, since American women tend to shave their underarms, ingredients are more easily absorbed into the skin, build up in the body, and then cannot be easily excreted by already compromised kidneys. Although, according to the article above, aluminum may contribute to Alzheimer's. Apparently, it builds up in the brain. Shows you what I know… or thought I know!

But then I found The American Association of Kidney Patients post from a 2008 article by Dr. Nathan Levin in *RENALIFE.*

"Most of the antiperspirants and some deodorants contain aluminum (Al), which is absorbed by the skin (Flarend et al – Food Chem Toxicol, 2001). In healthy people, it gets eliminated by the kidney, but for people with reduced function, Al will accumulate in the body. Albeit unusual, this could lead to dementia (Carpenter et al. – Int J Occup Med Environ Health, 2001), anemia and bone disease (Jeffery et al. – J Toxicol Environ Health 1996)."

So now we know the build-up of aluminum is also a problem. This goes right back to compromised kidneys not being able to eliminate the chemical that enters our bodies via the skin. Women are at risk since they shave their underarms which leave very small cuts in the skin, but men are also at risk. The chemical is applied to the skin, is absorbed, and builds up.

If you'd like to do more research yourself, take note that I got very few hits when I used 'Chronic Kidney Disease and deodorant,' but quite a few with 'CKD and deodorant.'

A Meta Is Going to Come? Shouldn't That Be a Change is Going to Come?

10/7/13 While I was debating whether or not it was time to take the flu shot all Chronic Kidney Disease patients are urged to take each year, the flu found me. No kidding about this compromised immune system business. I considered this a light case, but was just ordered back to bed... after over a week of laying low.

Keep in mind that this year's flu's vaccine only covers three or four of the many strains around, so you may end up with the flu even after having the shot. My family doctor's advice? Once you're well again have the inoculation and protect yourself from as many strains as you can.

I like that my new nephrologist is non-alarmist, non-paternalistic and easy going. When I told him that 50 as an eGFR reading was my panic point, he very gently reminded me that readings will vary within a range depending on the day, your hydration, etc. – all variable factors. I knew that.

Then he reminded me that after 35, we lose about 1% of our kidney function yearly. I was under the impression it was ½% annually and thought that started at a much later age. Finally, we talked about my reading of 48%. But I understood better now how that happened and am confident I can raise it again before I see him a year from now.

Enough about me, let's get to that metabolic syndrome. Oh, wait, that's about me too.

Kibow has sent me quite a bit of information about using their probiotics as a method of treating Chronic Kidney Disease. I need to warn you that this is not an endorsement of their product. I don't know enough about it yet.

Along with their press release, they sent me a booklet entitled ***Kibow's Educational Guide to Probiotics and Kidney Health*** written by Natarajan Ranganathan, Ph.D. and Henry D'Silva, M.D. In the booklet, they discuss metabolic syndrome. This part of that discussion lists five conditions in metabolic syndrome. Only three are necessary to diagnose the syndrome.

1. Abdominal obesity
 2. High blood pressure
 3. High blood sugar
 4. Low levels of 'good' HDL cholesterol
 5. High triglycerides

Except for the high triglycerides and low levels of 'good' HDL cholesterol, I have all these conditions. Granted, the abdominal obesity is self-diagnosed but you'd have to be blind to miss it.

So what's the big deal about metabolic syndrome? By the way, meta does mean change. According to The National Institutes on their Institute of Heart, Lungs, and Blood page:

"The term 'metabolic' refers to the biochemical processes involved in the body's normal functioning. Risk factors are traits, conditions, or habits that increase your chance of developing a disease."

The National Institutes is a fount of information on all topics that deal with your health.

Again, the same question: what's the big deal about metabolic syndrome? Usually it's stated backwards for Chronic Kidney Disease patients. The MayoClinic tells us,

"Metabolic syndrome is a cluster of conditions — increased blood pressure, a high blood sugar level, excess body fat around the waist and abnormal cholesterol levels — that occur together, increasing your risk of heart disease, stroke and diabetes."

Sometimes, Chronic Kidney Disease is mentioned as one of the diseases this syndrome puts you at risk for. We, however, already have that, so why should we try to either avoid the syndrome completely or ameliorate it if we do have it?

Before I was diagnosed with Chronic Kidney Disease, I joyfully proclaimed Dr. Andrew Weil as my health guru and actually had pretty good health following his suggestions. This is what he has to say.

"Doctors may also prescribe medications to lower blood pressure, control cholesterol or help you lose weight. Insulin sensitizers like Glucophage (Metformin) may be prescribed to help your body use insulin more effectively. It lowers blood sugar, which also seems to help lower cholesterol and triglycerides as well as decreasing appetite. The side effects of Metformin (often temporary) include nausea, stomach pain, bloating and diarrhea. A more serious side effect, lactic acidosis, can affect those with kidney or liver disease, severe heart failure or a history of alcohol abuse and is potentially, though rarely, fatal. Aspirin therapy is often given to help reduce risk of heart attack and stroke."

Notice the mention of kidney damage and that of aspirin therapy. We just can't take the chance.

Sometimes you just have to use your common sense. We *are* already at risk of heart disease, diabetes, and high blood pressure as CKD sufferers. Why would we take a chance of doubling our risk of developing these medical problems? Don't forget that while diabetes and high blood pressure can cause CKD, the reverse is true, too.

A Healthy Diet is Not Necessarily a Renal Healthy Diet

10/14/13 Many people have asked me why I just don't follow a healthy diet for my kidney disease. It's one of those questions we hear again and again as early stage Chronic Kidney Disease patients … and not just from those who think they know better, but from those who genuinely care about us and want to help. Today's blog is meant to answer that question.

There were many food guides from the government before the introduction of the one we usually hear about, the USDA's 1992 Food Pyramid. Although updated in 2005, this was the gold standard for a healthy diet. We'll be dealing with the 2005 revised version in this blog.

Michelle Obama changed all that in 2011 when she supported MyPlate as the new U.S. nutrition guideline in an effort to help control the obesity epidemic. By then, I was already on the renal diet so didn't really pay attention.

So what are the differences you ask?

Let's start with the base of the Food Pyramid which includes 6 oz. of bread, cereal, rice and pasta a day with the stipulation that half of these be whole grain. MyPlate suggests the same amounts. However, my renal diet considers a portion of pasta as 1/3 cup, not the 1/2 cup in the other two eating guides… however many calories a day I can eat.

That makes a difference because of the phosphorous and potassium CKD patients need to curb, to say nothing of our daily calorie limits. Even the protein adds up. For example, I'm limited to 60 grams of protein a day. That doesn't mean just meat. My favorite angel hair pasta has 7 grams of protein for a 2 oz. serving. Let's say I'd like half a cup. That's 4 oz. and already 14 of my 60 protein grams. Got to save some of those protein grams for the meat {turkey} balls!

Sometimes my 1200 calories seem like an awful lot, but not on the days I eat pasta or rice. You also need to keep in mind that the USDA bases their portion suggestions on a 2000 calorie diet. That means I, for one, will need to eat less food in each category and so will you if you don't require 2000 calories a day.

What about vegetables? Those are healthy, right? The 2005 Pyramid suggests 3-5 cups a day. I can't do that. MyPlate suggests 2.5 cups daily, but their cup for leafy salad greens is actually two cups. For the renal diet, one serving is 1/2 a cup. The government also recommends beans and sweet potatoes which CKD patients cannot eat due to their high phosphorous and potassium levels.   We need to stick to vegetables that are low carb and to limit or avoid salty ones.

Are you with me so far? The pyramid suggests two cups of fruit a day, while MyPlate suggests 2-4. That wouldn't be a problem except for the serving sizes which are different between these two and the renal diet. So no matter how healthy these are, I'm limited to three 1/2 cup servings a day. What does that look like? Today it was half a banana, 1/2 cup of blueberries, and one very small mandarin orange. As CKD patients, we need to be careful about {Yep, here it comes again.} phosphorous and potassium. As a matter of fact, bananas are a once in a great while treat due to their high potassium content.

Meat and Beans is a little bit of a joke since beans are a no-no for us. The pyramid suggests including nuts and seeds, too. Uh, not for CKD patients. Why? Because of the {You know it!} phosphorous and potassium. There's also the calorie consideration here. MyPlate has the same difficulties for us, although they suggest lean meat. We are urged not to have red meat too often and cheese – I know it's a dairy product – is included in our meat group. As renal patients, protein is not our friend with many of us being limited to 5 oz. daily. This group is where you get most of your protein.

Hang in there, almost done. The pyramid recommends 3 cups of dairy. MyPlate recommends 2 to 3 servings and they include cheese. {I find myself wondering if they mean real cups or MyPlate cups.} The most glaring difference is that the renal diet allows 1/2 cup of milk or plain yoghurt per day. I use a substitute since I'm lactose intolerant, but that's still only 4 oz. Why such drastic limitations? Tricked you. This time, it's not only the phosphorus and potassium, but also the sodium.

As far as oils, although nothing is mentioned about them on the actual plate for MyPlate, the pyramid does mention they should be used sparingly. The renal diet restricts them to 4 or 5 one teaspoon servings a day and is quite specific about which to use and which to avoid.

You do need to understand that this blog is based on MY renal diet for MY weight with MY restrictions at MY stage of the disease. Other CKD patients' diets will vary, but none of us can "just eat a healthy diet."

Psoriasis and CKD. These Two Things Go Together?

10/21/13   I have psoriasis. There, I've said {written} it. I'm now out of the psoriasis closet. Actually, it's so latent that no one would know if I hadn't just announced it – except for the thickening of one toenail – but there is a study that concerns me.

Last August, Dr. Joel M. Gelfand, Associate Professor of Dermatology and Epidemiology at the Perelman School of Medicine at the University of Pennsylvania in Philadelphia and his colleagues found that:

"...psoriasis was associated with an increased risk for nine diseases."

One of them is Chronic Kidney Disease.

For those of you who weren't sure, according to Psoriasis.com, psoriasis is,

"a chronic (long-lasting) disease of the immune system. While the exact cause of psoriasis is unknown, scientists believe the immune system mistakenly activates a reaction in the skin cells, which speeds up the growth cycle of skin cells."

There are seven types of psoriasis. The one you are probably familiar with – if you are familiar with any – is plaque psoriasis. WebMD tells us,

"About eight in 10 people with psoriasis have this type. It is also sometimes known as psoriasis vulgaris. Plaque psoriasis causes raised, inflamed, red skin covered by silvery white scales. These may also itch or burn. Plaque psoriasis can appear anywhere on your body...."

The word psoriasis is from the Greek psora which, appropriately enough, means itch. The outward manifestations are just that.

The current treatment is timed exposure to ultraviolet light, but that's only if topical treatment is not effective and before medication to ingest is prescribed. I'm being a bit vague here since each of the seven types requires a different treatment and each of those treatments varies based upon the severity of the disease the specific patient is suffering.

So much for background material. Now, about psoriasis and CKD. Researchers have seen this connection for some time, but it was never made as clear as it was in Dr. Gelfand et al's massive study which involved hundreds of thousands of all age adult patient records and questionnaires of those with mild and severe psoriasis, and controls {those without any psoriasis}.

On another note, some psoriasis sufferers do take drugs as part of their treatment.

What that means for us as CKD sufferers is that doctors now know they need to screen psoriasis patients for CKD, although it seems to be only those patients with over 3% of their bodies affected by psoriasis who have doubled their risk of CKD. With 60% of the population at risk for CKD, it could be that percentage may change once these routine CKD screenings for psoriasis are in place, especially since psoriasis is also so common among every ethnic group. This, of course, also includes those populations we know are at high risk for CKD.

Wow! Another way to save lives. Maybe we can lower that 50% of CKD sufferers who don't know they have it instead of allowing that percentage to rise. I know it's logical to think that more people who are screened will mean more people who have CKD {and that's true}, but these will be people who KNOW about their disease.

Just What The Devil Does Precancerous Mean?

10/28/13   Today, I received a call from the office of my dermatologist who just happens to be a soothing, easy to talk to doctor. They had the results of the two shave biopsies on suspicious lesions I'd recently had during my annual full body scan.

The second definition of lesion at The Free Online Dictionary is:

"A localized pathological change in a bodily organ or tissue."

The Mayo Clinic explains a shave biopsy, the kind I'd had.

"During a shave biopsy, the doctor uses a tool similar to a razor to scrape the surface of your skin."

My dermatologist wanted me to know the as yet still unhealed biopsy site on my right forearm was benign. Yay! But wait. The one on my forehead, the one I'd laughingly referred to as the hole in my head, was precancerous.

Just in case you need to know what happens to the biopsy material once it's been collected, according to WebMD,

"After the tissue is collected and preserved, it's delivered to a pathologist. Pathologists are doctors who specialize in diagnosing conditions based on tissue samples and other tests. (In some cases, the doctor collecting the sample can diagnose the condition.)

A pathologist examines the biopsy tissue under a microscope. By noting the tissue cells' type, shape, and internal activity, in most cases a pathologist can diagnose the problem."

I knew that and I knew what a shave biopsy was and I knew what a lesion was and I still felt my stomach drop. I also knew 'pre' didn't mean cancerous, but there was cancer in the word. We probably all know that 'pre' means before {from the Latin for prior}. Did that mean cancer was my inevitable future? Or my probable future if I didn't do something about it?

Split second decision on my part. "So, what do we do about that?" I asked, although I think I already knew the answer.

The procedure is called cryosurgery {I can't resist: cryo comes from the Greek for cold or frost. Perfect!} which my doctor's medical group defines as,

"the treatment of lesions with the application of a cold substance. In most cases, liquid nitrogen is used to destroy the lesion."

How did this happen? I'd had biopsies before but they were based on suspicious looking moles and were always benign. I needed a source I trusted, so I went to Johns Hopkins Medical Library. Oh, it was actinic keratosis we were dealing with this time.

What was that? This is their definition.

"Actinic keratosis can be the first step in the development of squamous cell skin cancer, and, therefore, is considered a *precancerous skin condition*. The presence of actinic keratoses indicates that sun damage has occurred and that skin cancer can develop."

I'm an optimist. Notice the CAN in the definition? That's what I'm banking on. That and the hope that my dermatologist can burn it all out so that it doesn't get the chance to develop.

As for squamous cell, I needed help with that, too. I found it at SkinCancer.org.

"Squamous cell carcinoma (SCC) is an uncontrolled growth of abnormal cells arising in the squamous cells, which compose most of the skin's upper layers (the epidermis). SCCs often look like scaly red patches, open sores, elevated growths with a central depression, or warts; they may crust or bleed. SCC is mainly caused by cumulative UV exposure over the course of a lifetime. It can become disfiguring and sometimes deadly if allowed to grow. An estimated 700,000 cases of SCC are diagnosed each year in the US, resulting in approximately 2,500 deaths."

The only risk factors I'd had were that I'd been fair skinned {I did notice my skin tone had darkened in the past decade since my move to Arizona} and I didn't wear a hat. I hadn't thought I needed one since my curly dark hair always tumbled over my forehead thereby – or so I thought – protecting it from the sun's rays.

I figured I'd better check this out to see if cryosurgery could have any effect on my kidneys. I doubted it, but then I hadn't known how dangerous the fluoride in toothpaste was either. I used the search term 'liquid nitrogen' since that's what will be used for the cryosurgery I'll be having.

While I may have scarring, there seem to be no indications that this substance enters the skin or blood stream much less that it exits the body via the kidneys. Can't exit if it never enters, right?

As for the scars, who cares? I already have a scar on my forehead from a previous shave biopsy in this exact spot about eight years ago. That one came back benign. Things change; be vigilant!

Testing...One...Two...Three...

11/4/13 On your mark, get set, test! Or not. It all depends upon which news articles you've been reading lately. You'd think it was a no brainer to automatically test for Chronic Kidney Disease when 60% of the U.S. population is at risk and more than 28,000 of those that do have the disease don't know they have it. That's what you'd think, but not necessarily what your doctors think.

Then there's the matter of "So what?" That's what I call reporting test results, but not acting upon them. According to The Clinical Journal of the American Society of Nephrology (CJASN)

"Automated eGFR laboratory reporting improved documentation of CKD diagnoses but had no effect on nephrology consultation. These findings suggest that to advance CKD care, further strategies are needed to ensure appropriate follow-up evaluation to confirm and effectively evaluate CKD."

That was more than a year ago. So much has happened since then. Yet, MedlinePlus, A service of the U.S. National Library of Medicine, National Institutes of Health posted an article from the American College of Physicians (ACP) which firmly suggests NOT routinely testing symptom free patients who have no risk factors while, at the same time, suggesting different methods for treating different symptoms at different stages.

For the only time I can remember, I ended up sitting in my office chair staring at my computer screen scratching my head in confusion after reading an article on this site. How can you treat what you don't know you have since you haven't been tested for it? To make matters worse, most of the early stages of CKD are *symptom free*. In this October, 2013, report, I found the following statement.

"There is no evidence that evaluated the benefits of screening for stage 1-3 Chronic Kidney Disease," ACP president Dr. Molly Cooke, said in a news release issued by the group. "The potential harms of all the screening tests — false positives, disease labeling, and unnecessary treatment and associated adverse effects — outweigh the benefits."

Wait a minute here, folks. I was diagnosed at stage 3 and have spent the last five years battling to stay in stage 3. Don't you think I'd rather be battling to stay in stage 1? Or even stage 2? You've got it backwards, Dr. Cooke. I'd rather deal with the labeling, the chance of a false positive, etc. and have caught this disease earlier so it never got to stage 3. I like living more than I do being label free, Ma'am.

Now for the other side of the coin. That same month, the American Society of Nephrologists (ASN) – which, come to think of it, is the first group whose articles I started reading when I considered writing a weekly blog – came out in support of routine testing calling CKD 'a silent killer.'

This is more to my liking. They talked about the chance to slow down, or perhaps even stop, the progression of the illness *once you know you have it* and the fact that the procedure is not only lifesaving, but low cost.

The National Kidney Foundation spokesman, Dr. Leslie Spry, had some interesting things to say about CKD in his Sept. 2013 blog in The Huffington Post.

"We, as a society, need to take kidney disease — which kills more Americans than breast cancer and prostate cancer combined — seriously, or the human and financial costs may become unbearable."

He was referring to both the approximately $60 billion dollars the government spends on treating CKD annually and the need for those over 60 to be routinely tested. According to Dr. Spry, too many people think of CKD as just something that happens as you grow older.

I know I didn't. Actually, I hadn't yet realized I was growing older. It was happening, but I wasn't paying any attention. It was the CKD – something I'd never heard of until I was diagnosed – that drove that fact home to me.

The whole purpose of the book, the blog, the Facebook page, and the tweets for **What Is It and How Did I Get It? Early Stage Chronic Kidney Disease** is to inform people about testing for CKD, and then becoming educated about the disease.

Bronchitis Veterans' Day

11/11/13 I've got bronchitis, so I went directly to The Mayo Clinic for a definition of bronchitis.

"Bronchitis is an inflammation of the lining of your bronchial tubes, which carry air to and from your lungs. Bronchitis may be either acute or chronic.

Often developing from a cold or other respiratory infection, acute bronchitis is very common. Chronic bronchitis, a more serious condition, is a constant irritation or inflammation of the lining of the bronchial tubes, often due to smoking.

Acute bronchitis usually improves within a few days without lasting effects, although you may continue to cough for weeks. However, if you have repeated bouts of bronchitis, you may have chronic bronchitis, which requires medical attention. Chronic bronchitis is one of the conditions included in chronic obstructive pulmonary disease (COPD). Treatment for bronchitis focuses on relieving your symptoms and easing your breathing."

That scared me. I did have bronchitis about six months ago, too, and both this time and last it hit hard. Yet I know that chronic is considered constant for at least three months and means

"long lasting, the opposite of acute"

Maybe this is just a case of two unrelated bouts of acute bronchitis. I did have a head cold just before the bronchitis. Alright then, if this is acute, or

"extremely painful, severe or serious, quick onset, of short duration; the opposite of chronic,"

why am I still having trouble breathing after three days?

By the way, both of these definitions are from the glossary in *What Is It and How Did I Get It? Early Stage Chronic Kidney Disease*.

I'm glad I have a follow up appointment with my family doctor on Wednesday, although I would have preferred one today.

WebMD tells us,

The symptoms of acute bronchitis may include:

- Hacking cough that persists for 5 days or more
- Clear, yellow, white, or green phlegm
- Absence of fever, although a low grade fever may occasionally be present
- Soreness in the chest

Okay, the disgusting green phlegm thing was there and the sore chest, but basically, I was having so much trouble breathing that I couldn't speak. This was not the scary asthmatic kind of couldn't catch my breath, but rather a having to work very hard to breathe.

So what brought me to the emergency room? My PCP {Primary Care Physician} is not in on the weekends and the Urgent Care Centers out here in Arizona made it clear they couldn't treat me because, as a CKD patient, I would need blood tests before any work could be done on me. Although, they ignored the blood tests at the emergency room long enough to give me a breathing treatment for which I am eternally grateful. I was still feeling miserable after it, but I could breathe a bit more easily. Ms.-I-Don't-Want-Medication did not even fight the need to use a nebulizer while I recovered. Let's just say I saw the value of breathing.

I'm also on an antibiotic since the cause {in my case} was deemed most likely bacterial and I do have CKD. Although the attending doctor said something odd, "Your creatinine is 1.2. We don't even consider that CKD." Why not? It's stage three.

I've heard this before. Apparently it goes back to that controversy about not diagnosing patients until they're end stage so they aren't living a label. Just in case you're interested, I think that's nonsense. If I'd been diagnosed earlier, maybe I could have maintained at stage 1 or 2, as I am at stage 3.

Easy, Peasy Cryosurgery

11/18/13   This is the feel good blog, the one to reassure you about a medical procedure. I have a friend who worries that my blogs scare people… and maybe they do, but they're meant to be informational – just informational. Except this one. This one is definitely meant to be reassuring.

With all the medical messes, we've had lately {She writes as her chest burns and a headache creeps in.} the solution to this one was the safest and quickest. The procedure to correct it is non-invasive, doesn't enter the body in any way, and – therefore – is totally safe for Chronic Kidney Disease patients.

I know, I know, slow down. Okay, from the beginning…

Skin cancer is responsible for almost half the cancer cases. According to the ***American Cancer Society's 'Skin Cancer Facts,'***

"It is expected there will be 76,600 cases of melanoma this year alone."

Melanoma, the most dangerous of the skin cancers, has made its unwelcome appearance in my family, so every year – well, it'll be every six months after this episode – I submit to a full body scan by my dermatologist. I say submit because I'm an old fashioned prude these days. However, she does manage to put me at ease each time.

During this last exam, she found something on my forehead… but it wasn't cancerous, just precancerous. That, of course, was enough to get me researching. Here's where I insert the usual disclaimer: I am not a doctor, folks, just someone with CKD who doesn't want to make her kidneys function even less effectively because she unwittingly had some medical procedure she shouldn't have.

What the dermatologist found is called actinic keratosis. This is also called solar keratosis and senile keratosis. I immediately latched on to the last name for this kind of precancer. According to HealthySkin.com,

"Senile keratosis is essentially a form of solar or actinic keratosis. However, the difference is that the senile form of this skin condition specifically refers to the elderly. Generally, this form of keratoses appears in individuals who are older than 50."

That's the second time in one week this 66 year old has been referred to as elderly. Oh right, don't get side tracked.

Solar, senile and actinic keratoses are the same precancerous condition. One thing that disturbed me about the information is that while I am light skinned - and so – prone to this type of precancer, it was on my forehead. Those of you who know me also know that I always have curls tumbling down across my forehead, including the affected area. This means it wasn't exposed to the sun and I avoid the sun at all costs anyway. This IS Arizona.

I was puzzled and dug further. MedicineNet must have been listening to me. This is what I found there.

"When patients are diagnosed with this condition, they often say, 'But I never go out in the sun!' The explanation is that it takes many years or even decades for these keratoses to develop. Typically, the predisposing sun exposure may have occurred many years ago. Short periods of sun exposure do not generally either produce AKs or transform them into skin cancers."

I do remember being talked into using aluminum foil to make a sun reflector so I could tan as a teen ager. I was so fair skinned that it never worked. Come to think of it, no one really knew about the ultraviolet rays of the sun/skin cancer connection at that time. Did they?

Ready to find out about this painless, quick, non-kidney threatening treatment? It was cryosurgery, which I've discussed before. The simplest definition is the one I found at WebMD.

"Cryosurgery is the process of destroying a skin cancer (lesion) by freezing it with liquid nitrogen. Liquid nitrogen is applied to the lesion using a cotton applicator stick or an aerosol spray."

While my dermatologist was done spraying the area, I asked her what was next. She started telling me I need to clean the area with soap and water, then pat it dry. I thought that was an odd answer and asked again. We both realized at the same time that there was no 'next' for this procedure. It was done.

Sometimes, there's a blister after the procedure. If so, I was to use an antibiotic ointment and perhaps a Band-Aid over the area until the blister dries. I may have a scar. Good, maybe it'll balance out all the scars on my arms {Carpal tunnel surgery, a crazy very big dog we had, bad attempts at food prep and ironing, etc.}. It may also remain white. Who cares? It is under my curls, as I've mentioned.

I never experienced the burning sensation or pain that others might in the first 24 hours. It, well, Spiderman tingled. Whoops! I think I'm aging myself again.

Down in the Mouth

11/25/13 With all that's going on here, I managed to add insult to injury... all by myself. While trying to open the jar of honey so I could sweeten Bear's tea, I broke my tooth. I was sleep deprived, still recovering from that terrible bronchitis and all I could think was, "Why didn't that hurt? I'm standing here with a piece my tooth in my hand and it doesn't hurt."

It took a few minutes for me to focus. That's when I realized it was not my real tooth; it was the plastic replacement for one of my two front teeth. I contemplated not having it fixed since it didn't look *that* bad. Ah, but I could hear the lisp when I spoke. I'd spent quite a bit of time in speech therapy when I was a youngster to lose the lisp and I didn't want it back again.

Hmmm, I've been trying to figure out how to whiten my teeth. People looked wonderful and really healthy with white teeth. I wanted white teeth, too, until I heard how much that would cost me. For vanity? No way, but now that it's a necessity....

I asked my dentist if I could get a lighter replacement bridge. I figured that since the bridge covered six of my top front teeth, the ones you see when someone smiles, it might be worth a shot. He agreed, so we'll go for the brightest available for the temporary bridge and see if the permanent bridge needs to be a darker hue. I find myself excited about this.

Here's what it has to do with Chronic Kidney Disease. I always urge you to speak to your doctor, every kind of doctor you have. That includes your dentist. I told him about my fear of pain in my mouth, the fear I've had since I opened a car door into my mouth at age 19.

That's what caused the need for the root canals in my two front teeth and the need to file them down, way down. I'd forgotten how very long they had been. I was warned the teeth might darken and flake in 20 years or so, but 20 years is a long time to a 19 year old.

They lasted longer than 20 years, but did eventually fall apart. That's when they were extracted and the bridge with the two new front teeth and anchors for two teeth on either side was inserted. That's probably a quarter of your mouth. Let's see you have 32 teeth and I had four wisdom teeth extracted which means 28 minus the one that… well, you get the point.

I asked for nitrous oxide, even though replacing a bridge is not a painful procedure. According to Medscape,

"nitrous oxide – commonly called laughing gas or sleeping gas – goes nowhere near the kidneys."

I remember researching when I first was diagnosed with CKD and calling my nephrologist to make certain it's safe. It is inhaled, goes into the lungs, and then is exhaled via respiration {breathing}. It doesn't go anywhere near the kidneys.

My dentist recognized that my fear was very real for me, assured me that nitrous oxide – which is combined with oxygen before you inhale it, by the way – would not be a problem and very gently asked me if I'd like something a bit stronger, say, valium.

Everyone's heard of valium, but I didn't know much about it and preferred not to take it. When I was in the throes of bronchitis {Was that only last week?}, the ER doctor wanted me to take cough syrup with codeine in it, but I'm really, really sensitive to drugs and knew that was going to knock me out. I didn't see the point and politely declined that, too. I'm not good with drugs.

So, valium. Can and do CKD patients use this drug? I found this warning in the Physicians' Desk Reference.

"Use Valium with caution if you have any type of kidney or liver problems."

There was nothing about WHY you need to be cautious in your use of valium. I spent an hour or more researching, but all I can find were admonition after admonition to tell your doctor if you have kidney disease and repeated mention that the dosage of the drug has to be accommodated to your degree of kidney function.

And (S)He's Safeeeeeeeeeeeeee

12/2/13 Having had no medical emergencies this past week, I was casting around for this week's topic when my dentist reminded me that I need to keep whitening my other teeth for at least another week so they somewhat match the new upper front six tooth bridge.

Whiteners... how do they affect the kidneys if they do at all? Should I use over the counter products? A kit I purchase from the dentist? An in-the-chair dental bleaching?

These are the kinds of questions I keep asking for deodorant, toothpaste, makeup, even waxing. Boy, have I ever covered a lot of ground in this area in the last couple of years. But, as usual, it's still not enough. I've been playing around with the idea of a newsletter based on what's safe and what's not as far as personal products and medical treatments.

I've already written about deodorants and toothpaste. What a response, especially to the deodorant blog! Most of my readers are not direct email, but read the blog via Facebook and that's where the lively discussions take place.

Here's another example. When I wrote about macular degeneration, I mentioned that my ophthalmologist offered his own designer vitamin that had a 25% chance of slowing down the sight loss involved in this disease. Once I eliminated the vitamins in the compound that were for preventing cataracts {I've already had those removed from both eyes}, I was still left with a bunch that might work and a doctor who didn't know what they would do – if anything – to my kidneys. I researched them one by one and discovered that only two would be safe for CKD patients.

Now, I don't mean to whine, but this is a lot of work for each new product you want to use. Sometimes even our nephrologists can't tell us because the product is so new. I've gone to the pharmacist with new products many times and, if they weren't too busy, they would call the company that made the product immediately. A call from a pharmacist seems to take precedence over a call from a consumer when it comes to inquiries.

I looked at the ingredients at the dental bleaching product I'd purchased and realized I would have to research them one by one. The dentist wasn't sure. The nephrologist was out of town and I didn't feel this necessitated a call from his covering doctor. The pharmacy was very, very busy. {We don't exactly have winter in Arizona, but we do have flu and cold season}.

There are nine ingredients in the dental bleach product I chose. One is water, so I didn't research that. I am not a doctor, never claimed to be one, and repeatedly reminded people that I am not one. Apparently, my computer hasn't gotten the message. But, while I am not a doctor, I'm a terrific researcher.

However, in this case, I could not understand even one of the articles I found about the eight ingredients I didn't know about. This was extremely frustrating. So, I did what I probably should have done in the first place: I called the company. They looked at the product information and assured me the product had no effect on the kidneys at all, but if I wasn't comfortable with that, to contact my local pharmacist and/or my doctor. I was willing to take their word for it, but I will call both the pharmacist and my nephrologist anyway. Just to be sure, you understand.

Ah, the problems of being a Chronic Kidney Disease patient... and we thought it was all about our doctors' appointments, diets, sleep, stress levels, and exercise!

'Twas The Night Before The Night Before Christmas

12/23/13 'Twas the night before the night before Christmas and all through the house…. The night before the night before Christmas? Where did the time go? Oh, I did know it was coming… just not so quickly.

And that's often the case when we deal with a chronic illness. We know that doctor's appointment is coming up and we're eager to see the results of our blood tests. After all, we've worked so hard on diet, exercise, sleep, and lack of stress {That's funny: stressing for lack of stress}. We just didn't know it was coming so quickly. Did we have enough time to lower our blood pressure? Was it enough time to lose some weight? Did we monitor our eating enough in this amount of time that our cholesterol numbers are down? Time, time, time. It all comes down to time.

I have a modest proposal {Apologies there, Mr. Swift}. What if we ignore time and just always – okay, almost always – watch the diet, exercise, sleep enough, and avoid stress? Oh right, that's what we're supposed to be doing: lifestyle changes.

According to an article published in the *European Journal of Social Psychology* way back in September of 2009, it takes an average of 66 days to form a new habit. The article was written by Phillippa Lally and her colleagues from the Cancer Research UK Health Behaviour Research Centre based at UCL Epidemiology and Public Health, and was based on their research.

Since it's habits that form your lifestyle, I had trouble accepting that number so I kept researching. Ugh, I kept coming up with the same number although one analysis of this same article did mention that it can take as few as 18 or as many as 254 days to form a habit depending upon the individual. I'll take the 18 days option, please.

All right, let's try something else. How about getting enough sleep. How much sleep is enough sleep anyway? According to Dr. Timothy Morgenthaler on The Mayo Clinic site, seven to eight hours is what an adult needs, but then he lists mitigating circumstances under which you might need more:

- **Pregnancy.** Changes in a woman's body during early pregnancy can increase the need for sleep.
- **Aging.** Older adults need about the same amount of sleep as younger adults. As you get older, however, your sleeping patterns might change. Older adults tend to sleep more lightly and for shorter time spans than do younger adults. This might create a need for spending more time in bed to get enough sleep, or a tendency toward daytime napping.
- **Previous sleep deprivation.** If you're sleep deprived, the amount of sleep you need increases.
- **Sleep quality.** If your sleep is frequently interrupted or cut short, you're not getting quality sleep. The quality of your sleep is just as important as the quantity.

When I was first diagnosed with Chronic Kidney Disease almost six years ago, the value of exercise was brought home again and again by my nephrologist. Until I researched for *What Is It and How Did I Get It? Early Stage Chronic Kidney Disease*, I wasn't clear about why this was important. This is what I discovered.

I knew exercise was important to control my weight. It would also improve my blood pressure and lower my cholesterol and triglyceride levels. The greater your triglycerides, the greater the risk of increasing your creatinine. There were other benefits, too, although you didn't have to have CKD to enjoy them: better sleep, and improved muscle function and strength. But, as with everything else you do that might impinge upon your health, check with your doctor before you start exercising.

I researched, researched and researched again. Each explanation of what exercise does for the body was more complicated than the last one I read. Keeping it simple, basically, there's a compound released by voluntary muscle contraction. It tells the body to repair itself and grow stronger. The idea is to start exercising slowly and then intensify your activity.

Okay, so we know during that 66 days to form a habit, seven to eight hours a night of sleep is one of the habits we should be forming and half an hour of exercise daily is another. Might as well throw in following the renal diet and avoiding stress as two other habits to get into.

Dragon in the New Year

12/30/13

I was trying to figure out what would be a good end-of-the-year topic
and kept getting the same vision of a heart. Unusual, I thought, since this
is not a feel good blog. In fact, it's sometimes downright scary. Then I
remembered that the heart pumps blood and there needs to be some
pressure for that. Of course! The last blog of 2013 would be about blood
pressure, a topic that's been bandied around quite a bit in the medical
field lately.

The year was new when Jane Brody of the New York Times wrote,

"48% of more than 76 million adults with hypertension have it under
control up from 29% in 2000."

That sounds terrific, especially since normal blood pressure was
considered lower than 120/80 at the time. But why is this outdated
information? Good question. Less than two weeks ago the 8th Joint
National Committee announced via the Journal of the American medical
Association {JAMA}, that the guidelines for hypertension {High blood
pressure} have changed. Keep in mind that hypertension can lead to
cardiovascular problems and kidney failure.

The new acceptable levels are 150 {Systolic} over 90 {Diastolic} for
people over 60. The big news for people with diabetes or kidney disease
– like us – who were considered to have hypertension at 130/80 is that it
has shifted to 140/90. This means that those of us who have been taking
hypertension medication because we have Chronic Kidney Disease and
were trying to stay below 130/80 can now go up to 140/90 without the
medication and as high as 150/90 if we're over 60. Personally, I don't
want to take the chance.

Apparently many doctors agree with me. Dr. Mariell L. Jessop, president
of the American Heart Association, says she's worried about public
reaction. As the medical director of the Pennsylvania Heart and Vascular
Center, Doctor Jessop said:

"I just get anxious when people hear that they don't need as much medicine and they can allow their blood pressure to drift up. But the American Society of Hematology {which means blood} and the international Society of Hematology have their own guidelines. According to these two groups, the acceptance of 150/90 for older patients should start at age 80, not 60."

There also seems to be a difference in the drugs that they recommend. These differences led the ASH/ISH authors to proclaim,

"Because of the major differences in resources among points of care it is not possible to create a uniform set of guidelines. For this reason we written a broad statement... and we expect that experts who are familiar with local circumstances will feel free to use their own judgment."

This does not add to my comfort at the thought of allowing my blood pressure to rise.

So here we have the first new sets of guidelines for acceptable blood pressure numbers since 1997 and they don't exactly agree with each other. Let's make matters worse for the layman. It also turns out that your blood pressure can vary as much as 20 degrees during the same day depending upon circumstances, food intake and the timing of that intake, and physical exertion. This actually makes a lot of sense to me.

The American Heart Association has a program called Heart360 in which patients send their daily blood pressure numbers to the health providers directly from their home blood pressure machines. 54% of the Heart360 home monitoring group reached their blood pressure goals after only six weeks as opposed to 35% of the group that was treated in the usual way: diagnosed, education about managing high blood pressure, and the importance of diet and exercise. While the first group received the same information, it seems to be the added monitoring that helped more people succeed.

Until next year,
Keep living your life!

Index

A
A1C, 21, 91-3
Aging, 60, 127

B
Blacks, 26, 72-4
Blood Pressure, See
Hypertension.

C
Carambola, See Starfruit.
Carbohydrates, 93-5
Coffee, 7, 60-1
Cryosurgery, 113-4, 119-21

D
DaVita, 7, 19, 24, 44, 48, 56-7,
    91
Degenerative Arthritis, 90
Dental Beaching, 124-5
Deodorant, 102-3
Diabetes, 43-8, 66, 72-3, 91-5,
    105-6
Dialysis, 30-2, 28-40, 56

E
Exercise, 34, 98, 127

F
Facebook, 40, 66-8
Flu, 8-14, 18-20, 104

G
Gall Bladder, 77-9
Gender, 64-5

H
Heat, 6-7

Heel Spur, 85-7
Hepatitis B, 57-8, 62-3
High Risk, 26-7, 36, 45-7
Humidity, 6-7
Hypertension, 19, 26-8, 36-7,
46, 128

I
Influenza, See Flu.
Inoculations. See Vaccinations.

K
KEEP, 30, 36-7
Kidney Diet, See Renal Diet.
Kidney Early Evaluation
        Program, See KEEP.

L
Lithium, 29-30
Liver, 57-8, 62-3, 78-9, 83-4, 96-
    8

M
Macular Degeneration, 80-2
Melanoma, 6, 119-21
Metabolic Syndrome, 55, 78,
        104-6

N
NAFLD, See Non-Alcoholic Fatty
        Liver Disease.
National Kidney Foundation,
        See NKF.
Native Americans, 48-9
Nephrology History, 31-2
Neuropathy, 99-101
Nigeria, 26-8

My Notes:

Have you read my other Chronic Kidney Disease books? Available on Amazon.com and B&N.com
(print and digital) or walk into a B&N to order them.

What Is It and How Did I Get It?
Early Stage Chronic Kidney Disease
SlowItDownCKD 2011
SlowItDownCKD 2012
SlowItDownCKD 2015
SlowItDownCKD 2016
SlowItDownCKD 2017

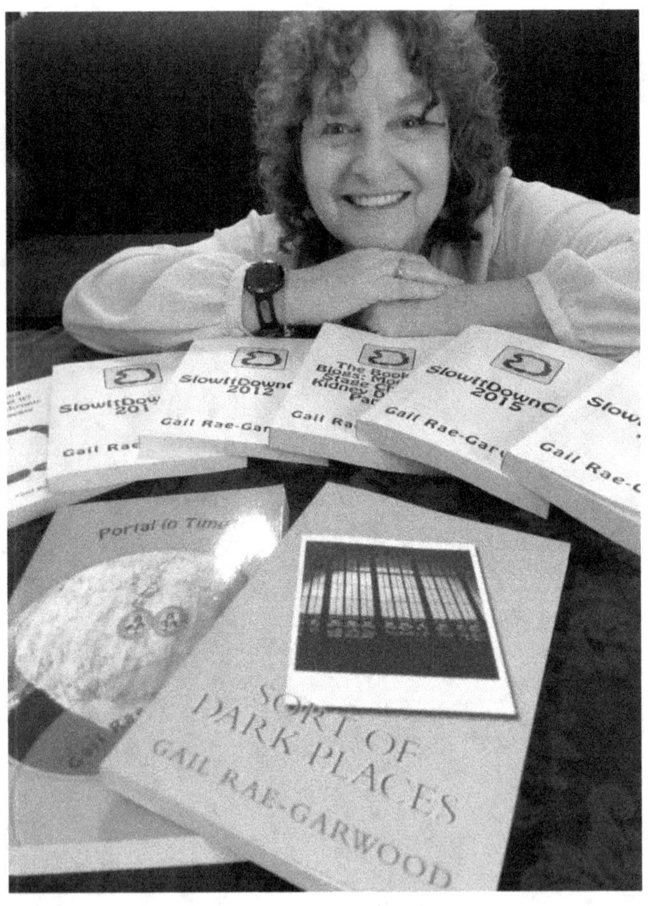

Follow the blog at
https://gailraegarwood.wordpress.com

SLOWITDOWNCKD

EARLY AND MODERATE STAGE CHRONIC KIDNEY DISEASE

On Instagram, Pinterest, and Twitter go to
@SlowItDownCKD

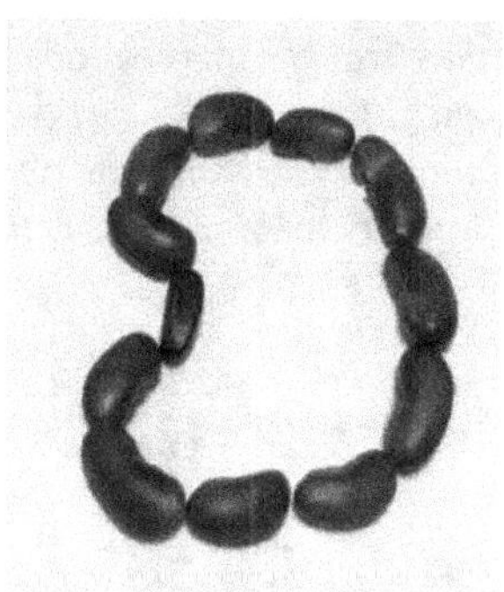

And then, there's the Facebook page at
*https://www.facebook.com/
SlowItDownCKD/*

Don't forget you can email me at
SlowItDownCKD@gmail.com

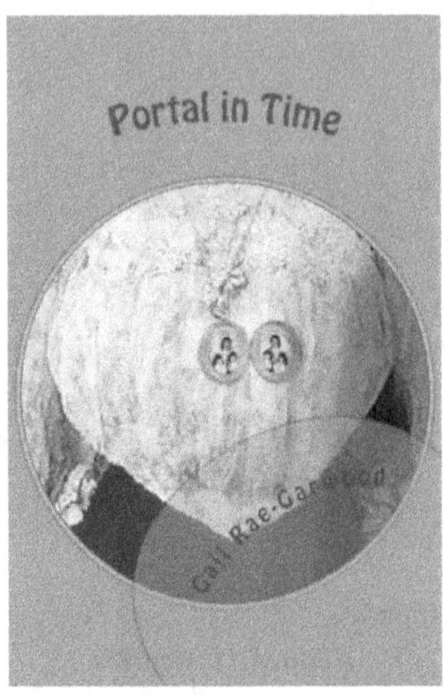

If you'd like to read a time travel romance (above) or fiction based on others' experiences (below), I've written one of each.
These are also available on Amazon.com and B&N.com
(print and digital) or walk into a B&N to order them.

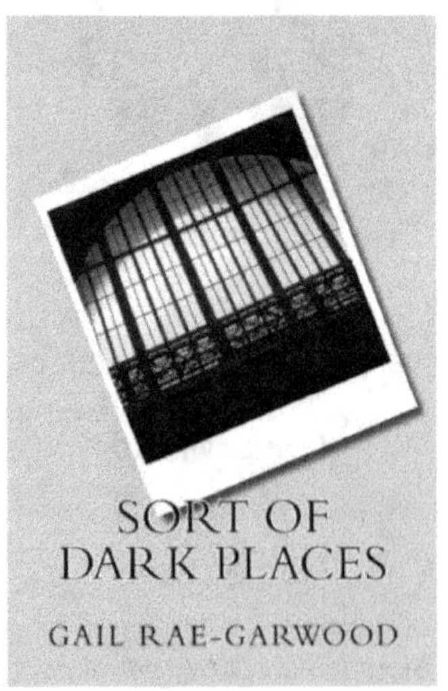

www.ingramcontent.com/pod-product-compliance
Lightning Source LLC
Chambersburg PA
CBHW070128260726

48658CB00001B/307